# THE DANIEL'S FAST

# COOKBOOK

Grace Bass and Lynda Anderson

The Daniel's Fast Cookbook

Published by A&B Publishing

Copyright © 2008 by Grace Bass and Lynda Anderson

ISBN: 978-0-9814768-0-3

Printed in the United States of America.

First printing: January 2008

Editor: Grace Bass

Proofreaders: Rev. Patrick W. Bass and Lynda Anderson

Webmaster: Rev. Patrick W. Bass

Art design (photographers): Grace Bass and Lynda Anderson

Cover Design: Grace Bass and Lynda Anderson

Sous Chef and Special Assistant: Lyle Anderson

This title is distributed by AtlasBooks Distribution.

# Disclaimer

The information contained in this cookbook, and its related websites, is provided for general informational purposes only. It is not intended as and should not be relied upon as medical advice. The information may not apply to you and before you use any of the information provided, you should contact a qualified medical, dietary, fitness or other appropriate professional. Recipes included in this cookbook are original. Any similarity with other recipes is unintentional. THE PUBLISHER AND AUTHORS MAKE NO WARRANTIES OR REPRESENTATIONS ABOUT THE ACCURACY OR COMPLETENESS OF THE CONTENT OF THIS BOOK OR ITS RELATED WEBSITES OR OTHER COMMUNICATIONS. INFORMATION CONTAINED HEREIN IS PROVIDED "AS IS" WITHOUT WARRANTIES OF ANY KIND, EITHER EXPRESSED OR IMPLIED, INCLUDING, BUT NOT LIMITED TO, THE IMPLIED WARRANTIES OF MERCHANT ABILITY, FITNESS FOR A PARTICULAR PURPOSES, OR NON-INFRINGEMENT OF THE RIGHTS OF THIRD PARTIES. THE PUBLISHER AND AUTHORS, THEIR AFFILIATES, DIRECTORS, OFFICERS, EMPLOYEES, SHAREHOLDERS, AGENTS OR ANY OTHERS INVOLVED IN THE CREATION OF THE WORK SHALL NOT BE LIABLE FOR ANY DIRECT, INCIDENTAL, CONSEQUENTIAL, INDIRECT, SPECIAL OR PUNITIVE DAMAGES RISING OUT OF ACCESS TO OR USE OF ANY CONTENT OF THE WORK INCLUDING BUT NOT LIMITED TO NEGLIGENCE, YOUR ACCESS TO AND USE OF THE BOOK, ERRORS OR INACCURACIES CONTAINED IN THE BOOK, EVEN IF YOU HAVE ADVISED THE PUBLISHER OR AUTHORS IN ADVANCE OF THE POSSIBILITY OF SUCH DAMAGE.

## Table of Contents

# Dedication

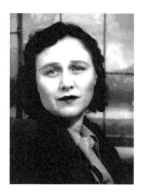

This Book is dedicated in the loving memory of our Grandma Fern.. Her love for God, family and friends was evident by the way she lived her life. Lynda's love for cooking was birthed at Grandma Fern's house. Grandma Fern always had a treat waiting...fresh strawberries from her garden or homemade cookies. If someone was ill, she was there with a meal. And each year she helped feed the threshers on the farms.

Both Grace and Lynda have fond memories of fishing with Grandma Fern. No matter how small your fish was, Grandma had a way of making you feel like it was a winner! She had a way of making you feel special. There is no doubt in our minds, that Grandma Fern is very much a part of the love and inspiration included in these recipes.

# About The Book

Many people are realizing the health and spiritual benefits of fasting. The Daniel Fast is just one of many types of fasts mentioned in the Bible. This book contains a thorough explanation of the Daniel Fast from a biblical perspective, as well as generally accepted guidelines for implementing it in your own life. The recipes in this book are based on what Daniel requested to eat to avoid being defiled. These recipes are purely vegetarian, whole grain and as close to the way God created it.

Some people desire to fast but cannot do a complete "water only" fast due to medical conditions. Others cannot go on an extended fast due to work or family obligations. Some will apply this fast as a lifestyle. There are others who recognize the health benefits and observe the fast strictly for the physical benefits. Whatever the motive, this book will help you draw closer to God while living a happy healthy life!

# What is The Daniel's Fast?

The Daniel's Fast is just one of the many types of fasts mentioned in the Bible. The fast described in this book is not EXACTLY the same as Daniel's original fast. It is based on what Daniel requested to eat to avoid being defiled when Israel was besieged and taken captive by Nebuchadnezzar king of Babylon.

When studying the scriptures, we first recognize the King's food was not compliant with God's dietary law established with the Israelites. Daniel's request to only eat "pulse" was to avoid breaking these laws- his intended purpose was to eat "kosher". The Daniel's Fast is a modified fast based on what Daniel avoided, not his intentions. Therefore, the Daniels fast is not simply a kosher diet (a diet following the Old Testament laws associated with food); it is a modified fast based on what Daniel requested to eat to avoid defilement.

Daniel 1:8 says *"But Daniel purposed in his heart that he would not defile himself with the portion of the king's meat nor with the wine he drank. Therefore, he requested of the prince of the eunuchs that he might not defile himself."* KJV

He did not eat meat or drink wine. Therefore, on the Daniel's fast there is NO meat or animal products.

Some people interpret "wine" in the Bible as fresh grape juice. But, I have a hard time believing Noah got naked on fresh grape juice. I am pretty sure it was fermented. Therefore, on the Daniel's fast I suggest avoiding all fermented products. (see Foods To Avoid for a partial list).

Daniel 1:12 says: *"Prove thy servants, I beseech thee, ten days; and let them give us pulse to eat, and water to drink."*

In simple terms, pulse is anything grown up from a seed. Barnes notes defines pulse as "what grows up from seeds-such, probably, as would be sown in a garden, or, as we would now express it, vegetable diet." Obviously, Daniel did not have all the variety we now enjoy. He was no doubt subject to seasonal fruits and vegetation of the region. I am quite sure he did not have access to filtered water either....We are not trying to duplicate his exact diet. But creating a modified or partial fast based on what he avoided and what today's "pulse" would be. Our modern day society of world trade, transportation and science has allowed us to enjoy a wonderful variety of foods year round. On the Daniels fast, we can enjoy this bountiful variety, while denying our flesh the "deceitful dainties" of this world.

During a Daniel Fast, I feel this is a time for spiritual cleansing as well as a physical cleansing. The typical American diet is full of processed foods containing many chemicals that pollute our bodies. The Bible says in Proverbs 23:3 "Be not desirous of his dainties: for they are deceitful meat." The "dainties" of this world are deceitful... they may look good, taste good and smell good.. but they are NOT good for YOU! I suggest avoiding all refined sugars (corn syrup, white sugar etc), white flour (striped, bleached and "enriched") and all products containing them. I also suggest avoiding all artificial sweeteners, flavors and colors, as well as additives, chemicals and dyes. These pollute and poison our systems. Hydrogenated oils are an "evil" of our modern day diet... you should avoid them all the time especially on the Daniel's Fast.

Hydrogenated oil is made by using a chemical process by which hydrogen is passed through heated oil. Completely hydrogenated oil becomes a solid fat. Partially hydrogenated oil is not completely saturated with hydrogen.  Thus, it becomes semi-solid in texture. Most butter substitutes are made of partially hydrogenated oil. It is relatively inexpensive therefore a majority of convenience foods available on our market place shelves contain partially hydrogenated oil. The American Heart Association and the American Diabetes Association both recommend reducing these from your diet. They have been linked to increasing cholesterol levels, obesity and diabetes among other associated risks.

One of the best alternatives to hydrogenated or partially hydrogenated oils is organic cold pressed oils.  Cold pressing is oil that has been made by pressing the seed, nut, olive, etc. to express its natural oil without the use of chemicals or heat. Many cold pressed oils are so healthy they are used medicinally. All cold pressed oils are "expeller pressed", however, not all "expeller pressed" are cold. In some of the hard nuts considerable pressure is needed to press out the natural oil. Heat is generated by the action of pressing. No external heat is used, therefore, "expeller pressed oils" are fine to use on the Daniel's Fast. The following page contains a partial list of cold and expeller pressed oils available.

Here is a partial list of cold and expeller pressed oils available:

- Olive Oil
- Brazil Nut
- Peanut
- Safflower
- Soya
- Sesame
- Sunflower
- Walnut
- Coconut
- Mustard Seed
- Macadamia Nut

In the Mediterranean diet, the Bible refers to olive oil frequently. When choosing from the many varieties of olive oils, cold pressed organic Extra Virgin olive oil is the best choice. It is the oil produced from the first pressing of the olives and is the least processed. Virgin olive oil is from the second pressing, Pure olive oil undergoes some filtering and refining, Extra Light olive oil has been through considerable refinement and processing- therefore it should be avoided on the Daniel's fast. Olive oil is high in antioxidants and is known to help protect against heart disease. Olive oil controls LDL(bad) cholesterol while raising HDL (good) cholesterol levels. It has also been linked to reduction of certain cancer risks.

# The Need

During one of my fasts, I searched for recipes for the Daniel's Fast but came back lacking. I ran into several people who also wanted recipes. I love cooking and soon developed many recipes that were compatible with the Daniel's Fast. My mother, Lynda Anderson, is a fantastic gourmet chef, so I asked her for help. She accepted the challenge with great humility and excitement! While working on recipes together, she told me she felt God had been preparing her for this very task all her life. Lynda shared an inspiring story from her childhood in Iowa about a harvest in which she helped feed the threshers. I have asked her to share it with all of you. The story is shared below. She is excited to know that all her knowledge of spices and cooking will be used to glorify God and "feed the threshers".

## *"Feeding the Threshers"*
### *By Lynda Anderson*

I remember my Grandma Fern making an apron for me when I was only five years old. She asked me to join her friends and help make food for the threshing crew. As in most small Iowa communities, harvesting the grain was very important. It was an event that many folks planned for all year long. I recall women bringing in canned jars from the bounty of their summer gardens. There were mason jars full of canned tomatoes and green beans. The fresh apples, so abundant in Iowa, provided for jars upon jars of apple sauce and apple butter.  At least ten women joined together with one purpose; to Feed the Threshers. Everyone worked together. A single combine served our rural community. It harvested and threshed the grain, which helped the laborers. Therefore, it was vital to help one another. The men dubbed Threshers would begin working before day break and return after dark. Men and young boys racing against time to bring the harvest in before it could be ravaged by nature. Families gathered and worked together to make sure that every farm would be harvested in time. In this we learned what love and sharing really meant.  From farm to farm the threshers would bring in the harvest. Everyone did their part. Women would work from sun-up to sun-down to provide as many as five meals a day.

As Christians we are commanded to pray for laborers. The Bible says *the harvest is plentiful but the laborers are few* Matthew 9:37-38.) As my daughter and I worked on recipes for this book, I felt as if I was somehow working again to Feed the

Threshers. Through fasting and prayer we help tear down walls and prepare the way for revival. True revival is a gift from God and requires us to work together with love and unity. As you go on the Daniel Fast and use the recipes in this book, I pray you are strengthened to work the fields.

# What the Bible Says About the Fast

*Daniel 1- KJV*

*In the third year of the reign of Jehoiakim king of Judah, Nebuchadnezzar king of Babylon came to Jerusalem and besieged it. 2 And the Lord gave Jehoiakim king of Judah into his hand, with some of the articles of the house of God, which he carried into the land of Shinar to the house of his god; and he brought the articles into the treasure house of his god.  3 Then the king instructed Ashpenaz, the master of his eunuchs, to bring some of the children of Israel and some of the king's descendants and some of the nobles, 4 young men in whom here was no blemish, but good-looking, gifted in all wisdom, possessing knowledge and quick to understand, who had ability to serve in the king's palace, and whom they might teach the language and literature of the Chaldeans. 5 And the king appointed for them a daily provision of the king's delicacies and of the wine which he drank, and three years of training for them, so that at the end of that time they might serve before the king. 6 Now from among those of the sons of Judah were Daniel, Hananiah, Mishael, and Azariah. 7 To them the chief of the eunuchs gave names: he gave Daniel the name Belteshazzar; to Hananiah, Shadrach; to Mishael, Meshach; and to Azariah, Abed-Nego. 8 But Daniel purposed in his heart that he would not defile himself with the portion of the king's delicacies, nor with the wine which he drank; therefore he requested of the chief of the eunuchs that he might not defile himself. 9 Now God had brought Daniel into the favor and goodwill of the chief of the eunuchs. 10 And the chief of the eunuchs said to Daniel, "I fear my lord the king, who has appointed your food and drink. For why should he see your faces looking worse than the young men who are your age? Then you would endanger my head before the king." 11 So Daniel said to the steward whom the chief of the eunuchs had set over Daniel, Hananiah, Mishael, and Azariah, 12 "Please test your servants for ten days, and let them give us vegetables to eat and water to drink. 13 Then let our appearance be examined before you, and the appearance of the young men who eat the portion of the king's delicacies; and as you see fit, so deal with your servants." 14 So he consented with them in this matter, and tested them ten days.  15 And at the end of ten days their features appeared better and fatter in flesh than all the young men who ate the portion of the king's delicacies. 16 Thus the steward took away their portion of delicacies and the wine that they were to drink, and gave them vegetables. 17 As for these four young men, God gave them knowledge and skill in all literature and wisdom; and Daniel had understanding in all visions and dreams.  18 Now at the end of the days, when the king had said that they should be brought in, the chief of the eunuchs brought them in before Nebuchadnezzar. 19 Then the king interviewed them, and among them all none was found like Daniel, Hananiah, Mishael, and Azariah; therefore they served before the king. 20 And in all matters of wisdom and understanding about which the king examined them, he found them ten times better than all the magicians and astrologers who were in all his realm. 21 Thus Daniel continued until the first year of King Cyrus.*

# It's Not All About the Food

## *Seeking God and "Taking out the Trash"*

Daniel's reason for abstaining from certain foods (fasting) was to keep from defiling himself (Daniel *1:8).* The Daniel Fast is not all about the food! If it were, the spiritual benefits of the fast would be negated. The result would be a life style choice on how to eat, or, simply put, a new twist on the vegetarian diet. This is a time to "Take out the Trash". Do an inventory. What consumes your time from God and Family?

What TV programs are you watching?

How much time are you surfing the internet?

What books are you filling your mind with?

Do they edify God?

During this fast you should consider turning off your TV. Don't watch movies, or read books that don't deepen your walk with God. Choose books on spiritual matters.  Spend more time reading the Bible and more time in prayer. Get off the Computer! I think we can waste just as much time surfing the internet as we do surfing the television channels.

## *Get your Priorities Straight*

During your fast you need to keep your priorities straight.

1. God- Prayer and Bible study
2. Family
3. Church and Community (serving Christ) reach out to your neighbor. Remember the parable... Who is your neighbor? This might be a good time for you to teach or prepare for a Bible study.

If you are fasting with your spouse, you may want to discuss the option of abstaining from sexual intimacy for the duration of the fast. This will enable both of you to "give yourselves more completely to prayer." You must BOTH agree.

1 Corinthians 7:5-6

*5 Do not deprive each other of sexual relations, unless you both agree to refrain from sexual intimacy for a limited time so you can give yourselves more completely to prayer. Afterward, you should come together again so that Satan won't be able to tempt you because of your lack of self-control.*

## What Kind of "Junk is in the Trunk"?

Envy, strife, anger, jealousy, lust, pride, laziness, depression, hostility, keeping record of wrongs (not forgiving) these things can easily take root in a person's life and hinder our relationships with people and God.

Galatians 5:19-23:

*"Now the works of the flesh are manifest, which are these; adultery, fornication, uncleanness, lasciviousness, 20 Idolatry, witchcraft, hatred, variance, emulations, wrath, strife, seditions, heresies, 21 Envyings, murders, drunkenness, revellings, and such like: of the which I tell you before, as I have also told you in time past, that they which do such things shall not inherit the kingdom of God. 22 But the fruit of the Spirit is love, joy, peace, longsuffering, gentleness, goodness, faith, 23 Meekness, temperance: against such there is no law"*

Let's dump the junk. Don't deceive yourself... truly search yourself. Ask God for help. Seek the Fruit of the Spirit:

Matthew 5:6:

*"Blessed are those who hunger and thirst for righteousness, for they will be filled."*

Remember, Daniel and his friends received some good things as a result of their dedication.

Daniel 1:17:

*"As for these four children, God gave them knowledge and skill in all learning and wisdom: and Daniel had understanding in all visions and dreams"*

Is there someone in your life you need favor with? Someone who has authority over you?

*"Now God had brought Daniel into favour and tender love with the prince of the eunuchs."* (Daniel 1:9)

There are benefits to fasting both spiritual and physical. When we fast we should keep in mind the scripture in Isaiah

Isaiah 58:6-10:

*"Is not this the fast that I have chosen? to loose the bands of wickedness, to undo the heavy burdens, and to let the oppressed go free, and that ye break every yoke? 7 Is it not to deal thy bread to the hungry, and that thou bring the poor that are cast out to thy house? when thou seest the naked, that thou cover him; and that thou hide not thyself from thine own flesh? 8 Then shall thy light break forth as the morning, and thine health shall spring forth speedily: and thy righteousness shall go before thee; the glory of the Lord shall be thy reward. 9 Then shalt thou call, and the Lord shall answer; thou shalt cry,*

*and he shall say, Here I am. If thou take away from the midst of thee the yoke, the putting forth of the finger, and speaking vanity;"*

If we fast with faith and the right attitude, we can expect good things to happen both in the spiritual and physical.

Becoming aware of the amount of junk you consume and the effects of that food is another benefit of the Daniel Fast. Our bodies are the temple of the Holy Spirit. As Christians we should be concerned with what our temple is made of. After all, we are what we eat. Here's a thought; If you were in charge of building the temple of God in the Old Testament would you use cheap wood, fake gold, and poor craftsmen? NO WAY! Only the best!!! We need to take care of our bodies: eat healthy food and exercise. Do the best that we can with what we've been given!

# Power in Prayer and Fasting

Before surrendering my life to Christ, my marriage was in shambles and my life was a mess. I hated my husband and was looking for a way out, but God continued to be patient and have mercy on me. After a very powerful experience in an altar, a friend gave me a book called "When ye Fast" by Joy Haney. After devouring the book, I felt a need to fast for my husband. I had never fasted before but I was desperate for a miracle. I went on a 21 day "water only" fast. It was extremely hard. My first 3-5 days were excruciating. I thought my head was going to split in two! I was a very heavy coffee drinker, therefore going cold turkey was very painful! At first my prayers were about my husband. "God change my husband...etc" soon they changed. Fasting had made me more sensitive to God. He was dealing with me and my part in our marriage. I had to swallow a lot of pride and I did a lot of crying. At the end of the fast, the hate that consumed my heart was replaced with a love that was not my own. I saw my husband with God's eyes. I loved him so deeply. Soon after the fast, my husband who hated God came to church was baptized and received the Holy Ghost! Our new life in Christ began. I really believe this fast broke spiritual bands and helped us both break free.

I have been on many fasts since this first one. I can say with absolute certainly, fasting will make you more sensitive to God. It helps clean out the cob webs... whether it's an absolute fast or a partial fast (such as the Daniel Fast), God honors your faith.

## *Corporate Fasting:*

The Daniel fast is a great fast to go on as a church body! I have attended a church that goes on a Daniel Fast for 40 days every year!! The results are amazing! The Church Body binds together in prayer and fasting which promotes unity! Many amazing things have happened, hearts have become more tender, relationships restored, lives have been changed, healings and deliverance! If your church is ready to storm the gates of hell, come together in unity..fast and pray together!

# Frequently Asked Questions

## How long should I fast?

Daniel started the fast with a ten day test. Likewise, many people make a ten day commitment to the fast. After Daniel and his friends passed the test they were allowed to continue on the fast indefinitely. Keeping this in mind, the duration of your fast is between you and God. However, keep your commitment. If you say you are going to fast for ten days, don't stop at nine.

## What did Daniel feel would defile him?

Well, the king's food was against the dietary laws God had previously established with the Israelites. Daniel and his friends also vowed against the wine most likely because it had been offered to idols. We also know the meat was offered up to idols/demons.

## What is Pulse?

In simple terms, pulse is anything grown up from a seed. Barnes' Notes defines pulse as "what grows up from seeds - such, probably, as would be sown in a garden, or, as we would now express it, vegetable diet." The application of the pulse or "vegetarian" diet has a broad spectrum. I have heard of people who apply this very liberally to include processed foods, fast foods such as French Fries from McDonald's and dairy like butter, cheese, milk, etc. They basically abstain from meat. Some food items you will need to ask yourself, "Is this a king's dainty?"

As I have mentioned before, I feel this is a time of spiritual cleansing as well as a physical cleansing. It should cost your flesh something. The typical American diet is full processed foods containing many chemicals that pollute our bodies. Therefore, processed food should be avoided. I also promote the use of organic foods. The closer to the way God created it the better.

1Barnes' Notes, Electronic Database. Copyright (c) 1997 by

Biblesoft

# Guidelines: Foods to Avoid

- ALL meat product including sea food, beef and chicken broth, etc.
- Imitation meat products (artificially flavored, highly processed)
- Dairy products such as milk, cheese, sour cream, etc
- All egg products
- Grains that have been bleached and processed such as white flour and all products containing it
- White sugar and all products containing it
- White rice
- Artificial Sweeteners (Splenda® (sucralose), NutraSweet® (aspartame), Sweet'N Low® (saccharine), etc.)
- Carbonated beverages (soda, soft drinks, carbonated flavored water, etc)
- Foods containing additives, chemicals and dyes
- Soy sauce (fermented)
- Artificial anything including flavors and colors
- Hydrogenated oils (margarine, shortening and all products containing it)
- Fried food should be avoided (most fried foods are fried in Hydrogenated oil)
- Corn Syrup (high fructose corn syrup)
- Alcohol - Daniel didn't drink the king's wine
- Vinegar - made by a fermentation process like wine
- Black Tea- fully fermented
- Baking powder - it is baking soda (natural) and an acid like cream of tartar mixed together. Cream of tartar is a byproduct of wine making.
- Caffeine*
- Yeast*

*See foods for personal conviction

# Guidelines: Foods to Enjoy

- All fruits and vegetables- fresh, frozen dried or canned
- All grains, beans, legumes, that have not been bleached stripped and processed. Grains should be whole. Such as whole brown rice, whole wheat flour etc.
- All nuts
- All herbs and seasonings and spices -salt is fine. Try and use natural herbs and seasoning
- Baking soda- all natural
- Agave Nectar- this is great! It is all natural and has a consistency similar to honey... just a little thinner. PLUS- the glycemic index of Agave nectar is VERY low.
- Stevia (for more information see page 40)
- Bragg Liquid Aminos® (natural alternative to soy sauce)
- Water, naturally decaffeinated tea, fruit and vegetable juices
- Cold pressed oils such as olive oil, unprocessed coconut, peanut, sesame, walnut, almond, and mustard seed oil
- Soy Milk (read the nutritional label)
- Tofu (whole soy beans and water)
- Pasta (whole-grain flour and water) NO EGGS or WHITE flour
- Honey*
- Maple syrup*
- Raw cane sugar*

*See foods for personal conviction

# Foods for Personal Conviction

## Yeast

Yeast is not an animal product nor is it a man made chemical. In baking and cooking yeast is used as a leavening agent, where it converts the fermentable sugars present in the dough into carbon dioxide. This causes the dough to expand or rise as the carbon dioxide forms pockets or bubbles. When the dough is baked it "sets" and the pockets remain, giving the baked product a soft and spongy texture. Because of the fermentation involved, many people will choose to avoid yeast during a Daniel Fast.

## Caffeine

Caffeine is an addictive substance. Therefore, it can become a weight in the walk of a Christian. It may be a good idea to detoxify your body by abstaining. However, I am aware of people with medical conditions that fight EXTREME fatigue. In such instances, caffeine is often used for its medicinal purposes to help energize the body. If you choose to use caffeine during a Daniel Fast you should still abstain from cow's milk, cream, non-dairy creamer, sugar, artificial sweeteners and syrups.

## Grapes, Raisins, or Grape Juice

Some people interpret "wine" in the Bible as fresh grape juice. But I have a hard time believing Noah got naked on fresh grape juice; I am pretty sure it was fermented. The reason Daniel didn't want to drink the king's wine was because it was offered to idols. If we follow this train of thought, we will be defining the Daniel Fast as a Kosher diet (eating all foods that follow Old Testament dietary law). In essence, this is what Daniel was trying to comply with. In contrast, however, this is not the intention of the modified fast. As I mentioned before, this isn't the exact diet Daniel ate but based on what he requested to eat Pulse...food grown from a seed. Daniel didn't want to eat the king's meat or drink the king's wine. Therefore, this fast avoids all animal products, fermented substances, and allows all things grown from the ground. In my opinion, grapes, raisins and unfermented grape juice are fine.

## Natural Sweeteners

*Honey, maple syrup and natural raw sugar cane*

Honey is made by bees out of flower nectar. It is not really considered vegan, because it is a product of a living being. The decision to allow honey on your Daniel fast is between you and God.

*Maple syrup*

Maple syrup is made from the sap of maple trees. It is then boiled down until enough water has evaporated to make syrup. Maple syrup is all natural, it is not a product of an animal and it has not been tainted by man with chemicals. Therefore, I think using Maple syrup is ok on the Daniel fast. However, some people will avoid all sugar/sweets on the fast.

*Raw sugar cane*

Sugar Cane is grown from a seed. However, it goes through a considerable amount of processing. Refined white sugar is definitely not Daniel Fast friendly. True raw sugar is better than white refined. If you choose to allow it on your fast, use it sparingly.

*Judge for Yourself*

Two questions you can use as a general rule of thumb: Did it grow from a seed? Has man polluted it? Has it been fermented? If you can answer these questions with any degree of certainty then you can be reasonably assured that your food choices are in line with The Daniel Fast.

# Reading Nutritional labels

During one of my fasts, I needed a snack while I was out running errands. I stopped at a health food store and purchased a health bar. The health bar had an attractive wrapper proclaiming 100 % vegetarian, dairy free, organic, live whole grains. It looked perfect! As I was driving, I bit into the bar, it was so nasty! But, I was hungry and thought, "it taste bad, it MUST be good for me!" When I stopped I became curious about what made it taste so awful, so I read the ingredients. It was loaded with FERMENTED grains and fruit! UGGG I was very upset. I learned right then and there: ALWAYS read the list of ingredients.

Once I began reading the ingredients on the foods I consumed, I was shocked at the amount of chemicals and unhealthy junk I put into my body. For instance, most bread that can be purchased at the store contains hydrogenated oils, refined sugars and other items listed on the "foods to avoid list". Be aware that "multi-grain" doesn't mean "whole grain".

# Nutritional Concerns

*Protein*

Protein is the building blocks of our bodies, it is necessary for life. Many people have concerns about consuming enough protein when they abstain from all meat and animal products. The Recommended Daily Allowance (RDA) recommends we consume 0.8 grams of protein for every kilogram (or .36 grams of protein per pound) we weigh.

- Body weight (in pounds) x.36= recommended protein intake

For example, if you weigh 145pds the formula would be

145 pds X .36 = 51.7 grams of protein

Consuming this amount of protein is not difficult on the Daniels fast. Protein can be found in nearly all vegetables, beans, grains, nuts and seeds. As long as you consume a variety of whole unrefined grains, legumes, seeds, nuts and vegetables though out the day, you will probably get enough protein.

## Calcium

Dairy products are not allowed on the Daniel's Fast. Many Americans believe dairy products are the primary source of calcium in our diets. However, calcium is abundant in leafy green vegetable as well as some fruit, beans and grains. Although you may be able to meet your daily intake goals eating these calcium rich foods, you may want to take a vegan all natural calcium supplement.

## B-12

Taking a B-12 supplement is especially important while on the Daniel's fast. B-12 is produced by bacteria. It is not in any animal or plant sources, unless they have been contaminated by microorganisms.

## Supplements

Before taking any new supplements please speak to your doctor. I recommend taking a vegan multi-vitamin, b-12 sublingual tablet and vegan calcium supplement. With careful meal planning you may be able to meet all your dietary needs while on the Daniel's fast. However, for those of you who do not have the time to study the vitamin/nutritional content of all fresh fruits, vegetation, nuts, etc. allowed on the Daniel's fast simply take a multi- vitamin to cover all your bases.

## *Garlic*

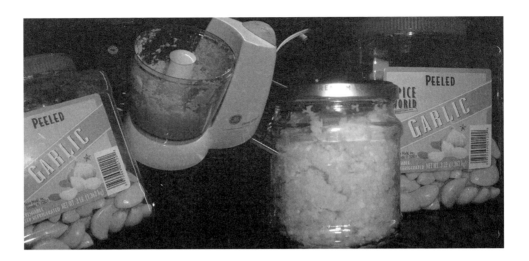

Many of the recipes in this book contain chopped garlic. If peeling garlic seems like a tedious task, here is a simple solution. Purchase fresh peeled garlic in the vegetable section at most super markets. As pictured above, simply fill your food processor with the peeled whole garlic and add 3 tablespoons of olive oil for every cup of whole garlic. Pulse the processor until reaching a "chopped" consistency. Store in a glass jar; will keep refrigerated several weeks.

# Daniel's Fast Friendly Restaurants, Stores and Products

Fasting while at work can be a challenge. Many people have mandatory lunch meetings or get caught up in the hustle and bustle and forget to pack a "Daniel fast friendly" lunch. This can be challenging, being in a restaurant that serves all the foods you love will test your resolve! Here are a few suggestions. Make a Daniel fast friendly salad dressing from the recipe section and carry it with you in a small container. Most restaurants serve salad, even McDonalds has a salad to choose from...just ask them to leave off the meat. If you forgot your salad dressing ask for lemons and squeeze fresh lemon juice over your salad, add salt and pepper to taste. Other ideas include ordering a baked potato and steamed vegetables. Make sure you ask them to hold the butter, sour cream etc. Just get the potato.

There are a few chain restaurants with Daniel Fast friendly menus. Chipotle, Qdoba Mexican Grill, Subway, and Cousins Subs. Applebee's has a steamed vegetable plate and a sizzling vegetable skillet (remember, no butter). P.F. Changs, Wendy's (Baked Potato) also offer good choices. Taco Bell does not use lard and so their refried and pinto beans are acceptable. Taco Bell's corn tortillas are ok as well. If you have any questions you can call them at 1-800-TACO-BELL, they seem very helpful.

Chipotle has a website with a wealth of information regarding their ingredients: www.chipotle.com their ingredients are organic and many of the items on their menu are Daniel Fast friendly.

# Products that are Daniel Fast Friendly

## *Stevia*

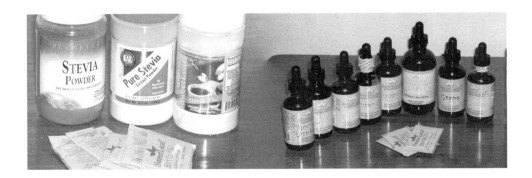

Stevia is a leaf that is naturally sweet. It is up to 300 times sweeter than sugar and has ZERO calories and ZERO carbohydrates. According to an article published in Low Carb Living, Stevia was first discovered by M.S. Bertoni and introduced to Europe in 1899. However, the Guarani Indians of Paraguay had been using the stevia leaves for over 1500 years. In recent years, it has become the dominate commercial sweetener in Japan. Not only is it a natural means to reduce or replace sugar without all the chemicals, it's good for you! Hundreds of scientific studies have been done on Stevia, and scientists are reporting numerous health benefits. Wisdom Natural Brands www.sweetleaf.com Offers a Stevia product that is great! They make Stevia powder in small packets (Sweet Leaf). I have purchased these from Wal-Mart and most health stores.  My local grocery store also carries it. Wisdom also produces liquid Stevia. It does not contain any alcohol and is Daniel Fast friendly. It comes clear and in many flavors: Vanilla crème, Cinnamon, Lemon, Valencia Orange, English Toffee, Milk chocolate, Dark Chocolate, Peppermint, Apricot Nectar, Root Beer and Chocolate Raspberry. The liquid Stevia is a little harder to find. I have ordered it from Wisdom's website and I have found it in Health food stores. Whole foods carried them all.

To Substitute 1 Cup Sugar use one of the following:

- 1/3 to 1/2 Stevia extract powder
- 1 teaspoon clear liquid
- 1 Tablespoon concentrated (water based)
- 1 1/2 to 2 Tablespoons ground or cut leaf
- 1 1/2 to 2 Tablespoons powder with filler
- 18 to 24 individual packets
- 2 teaspoons concentrated (water based)

## Bragg Liquid Aminos

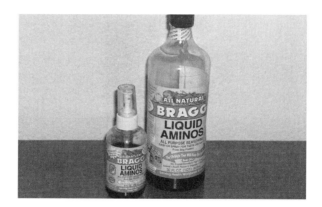

Bragg Liquid Aminos is distributed by Bragg Live Good Products www.bragg.com. This is a product made with vegetable protein from soybeans and purified water. It tastes like soy sauce but has not been fermented. Soy sauce is not Daniel Fast friendly because it is made by fermentation.

# Necessary Cooking Tools

**Food Processor**: An inexpensive one will do.

**Vidalia Chop Wizard**: Costs about $20. I have seen them at Target, Wal-Mart and my local grocery store. You can also order it on line at www.chopwizard.com.

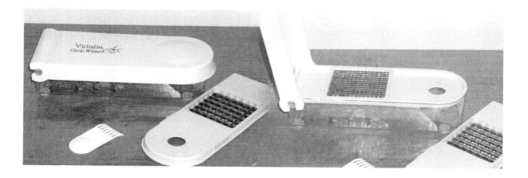

**Tortilla press:** They should cost around $20 I have seen them at World Market. I purchased mine on the internet at www.drillspot.com.  The service was great and shipping was fast.

# RECIPES

# Breakfast & Breakfast Breads

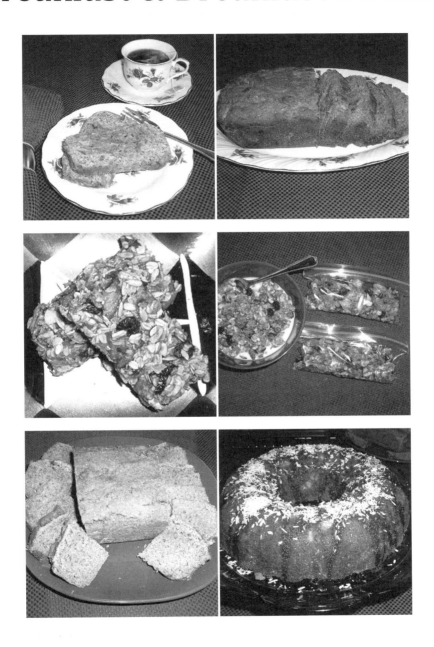

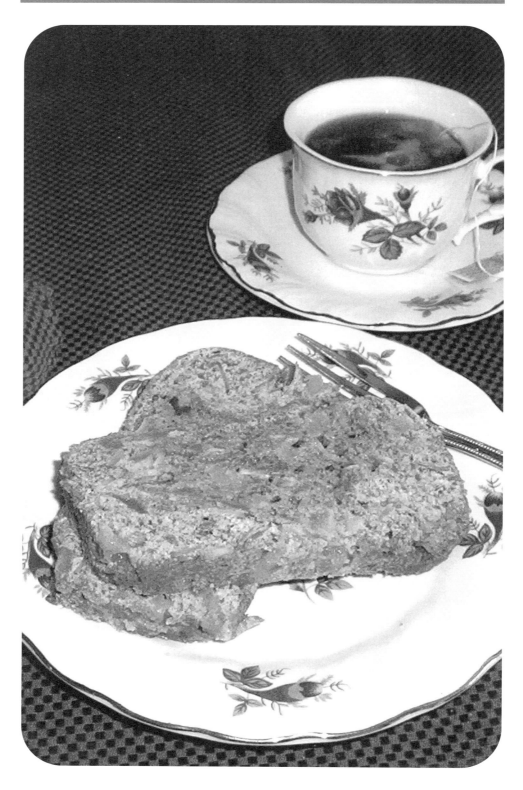

# Apricot Breakfast Bread

*1* teaspoon coconut oil, organic extra-virgin cold pressed for
   pan
*1 ½* cups dried apricots, cut into small pieces
*1 ½* cups orange juice
*2 ½* cups whole-grain wheat flour
*1* teaspoon baking soda
*1* teaspoon salt
*1* teaspoon cinnamon
*2* tablespoons coconut oil, organic extra-virgin cold
   pressed
*1/2* cup Agave nectar
*1/2* cup banana, mashed
*1* tablespoon orange zest
*1* cup almonds, sliced

### Instructions

- Preheat oven to 325°, grease loaf pan with coconut oil
  and lightly flour.
- In a small pot, bring diced apricots and orange juice to a
  boil.  Then reduce heat and simmer for 10 min.
- Combine wet ingredients in a large bowl: Coconut oil,
  agave nectar, mashed banana.
- In a separate bowl combine dry ingredients: flour, soda,
  salt, cinnamon and orange zest, mix well.
- Add dry ingredients to wet ingredients, stir in apricots
  with the orange juice and the sliced almonds. Stir until
  all ingredients are mixed well.
- Pour into floured bread loaf pan and bake at 325° for
  30-40 min. Cool on a rack.

**Recipe Notes**

*Test kitchens have noted a 25˚ to 50˚ temperature difference in ovens. Because of this temperature difference, it will be important for you to check your bread 5 to 10 min before the directions indicate it is done. Insert a toothpick in the center of the loaf, if it comes out clean the bread is done.*

*If possible use a glass bread pan. A dark pan may make the bread brown prematurely.*

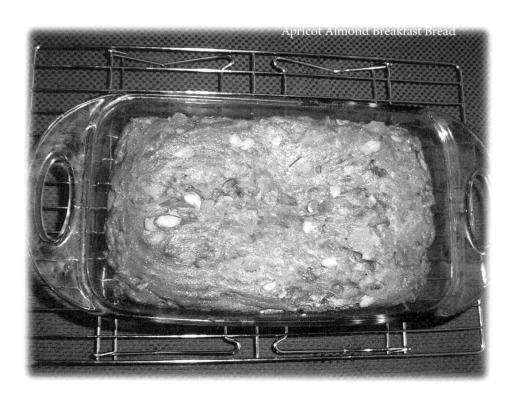
Apricot Almond Breakfast Bread

# Pumpkin Bread

*2* cups whole grain, whole wheat flour
*1* teaspoons baking soda
*1* teaspoon salt
*1* teaspoon cinnamon
*1/4* teaspoon all spice
*1/2* cup coconut oil, organic extra-virgin cold pressed
*3/4* cup raw agave nectar
*1* tablespoon lemon juice
*1* 15 oz. can pure pumpkin
*1* teaspoon coconut oil, organic extra-virgin cold pressed to
  lightly oil pan

### Instructions

- Preheat the oven to 350°.
- Use a 1 teaspoon of coconut oil to lightly grease the bread pan, then lightly flour.
- In a large bowl combine the agave and coconut oil. If the coconut oil is solid, melt in the microwave prior to mixing with the agave.
- In a small bowl combine pumpkin and lemon juice. Add to the agave mixture.
- In another small bowl combine flour, baking soda, salt and spices. Add to the agave, pumpkin mixture and mix well.
- Pour into bread pan and bake for 45min

### Recipe Notes
*Test kitchens have noted a 25˚ to 50˚ temperature difference in ovens. Because of this temperature difference, it will be important for you to check your bread 5 to 10 min before the*

*directions indicate it is done. Insert a toothpick in the center of the loaf, if it comes out clean the bread is done.*

*If possible use a glass bread pan. A dark pan may make the bread brown prematurely.*

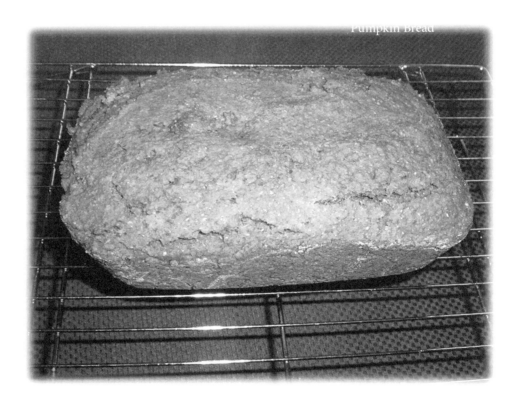

Pumpkin Bread

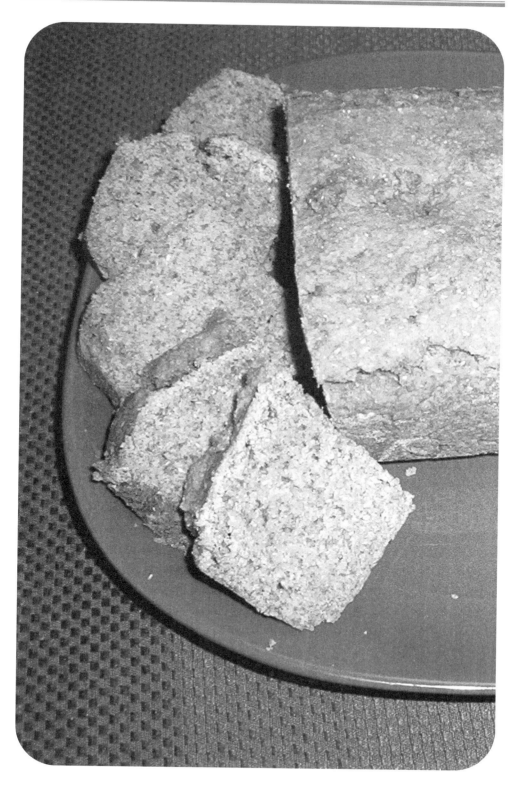

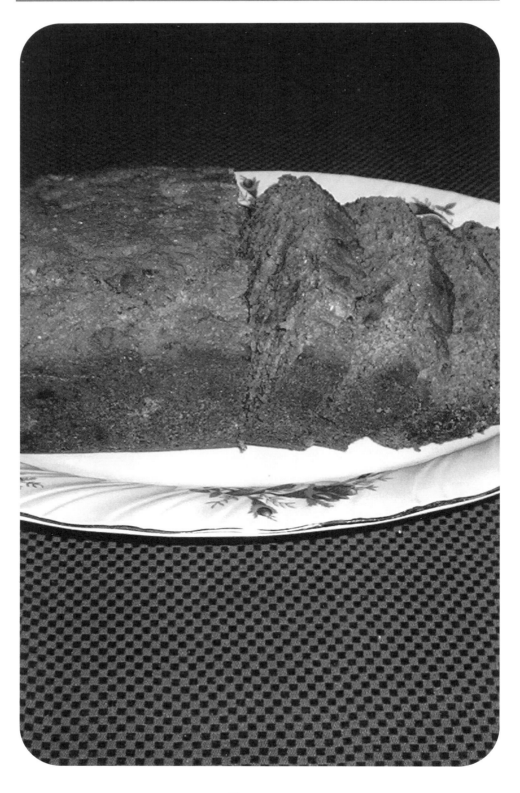

# Banana Brea[

*1* teaspoon coconut oil, organic extra-virgin co[
   the bread pan
*1/2* cup coconut oil, organic extra-virgin cold pres[
*3/4* cup agave nectar
*2* cups bananas, mashed
*1* tablespoon lemon juice
*2* cups whole grain, whole wheat flour
*1* teaspoon salt
*1* teaspoon baking soda

## Instructions

- Preheat the oven to 350°. Use 1 teaspoon of coconut oil to lightly grease the bread pan, then lightly flour.
- In a large bowl combine the agave and coconut oil. If the coconut oil is solid, melt it in the microwave prior to mixing with the agave.
- In a small bowl combine mashed bananas and lemon juice. Add to the agave mixture.
- In another small bowl combine flour, baking soda, and salt. Add to the agave banana mixture and mix well.
- Pour into pan and bake for 55min.

## Recipe Notes

*Test kitchens have noted a 25° to 50° temperature difference in ovens. Because of this temperature difference, it will be important for you to check your bread 5 to 10 min before the directions indicate it is done. Insert a toothpick in the center of the loaf, if it comes out clean the bread is done.*

*If possible use a glass bread pan. A dark pan may make the bread brown prematurely.*

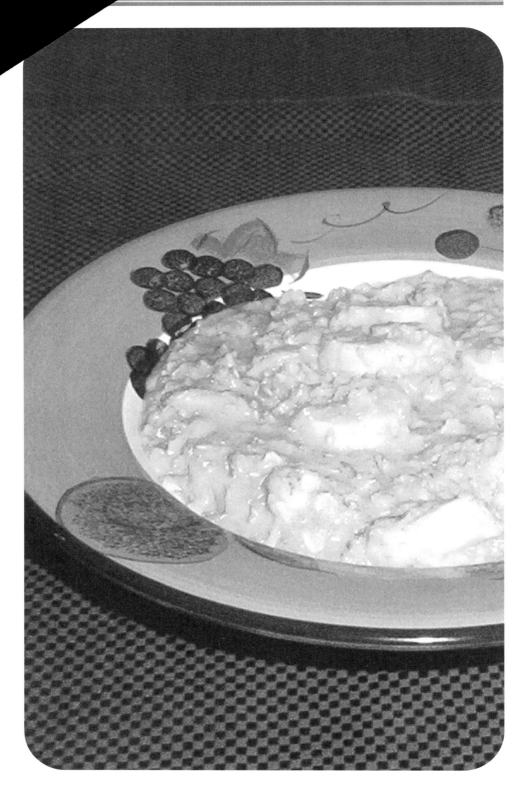

# Creamy Banana Oatı

*2* cups oats (Old Fashioned)
*3* cups Silk Organic Soy Milk (vanilla)
*1* whole banana
*1/4* teaspoon of cinnamon

### Instructions

- Combine Oats and soy milk in a medium pot. Cook over medium heat stirring continually until thick. Be aware that old fashioned whole oats take time to soften and thicken.
- Add fruit. I like using one banana. You may add agave to sweeten, however, I think the fruit makes it sweet enough.

### Recipe Notes

*When choosing a soy milk, make sure it's ingredients are ALL natural. I have found a few brands that add a lot of junk..*

Serves: 2.

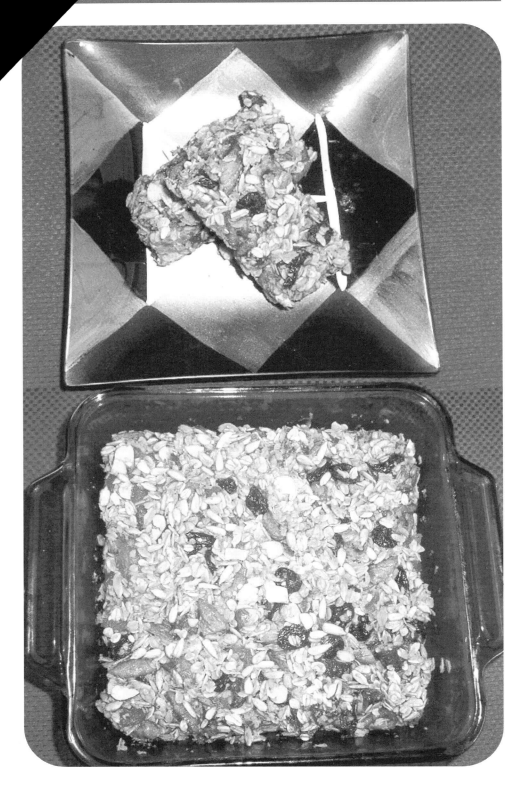

# Dried Fruit Bar

*1* cup agave nectar
*2* tablespoons peanut oil
*1* tsp of cinnamon
*1 1/2* cups oats (Old Fashioned), uncooked
*1/2* cup whole grain, whole wheat flour
*1/2* cup sliced Almonds
*1/2* teaspoon salt
*2/3* cup sunflower seed, salted
*10* whole dried apricots, cut in 5 pieces
*10* whole dried figs, cut in 5 pieces (make sure you cut off
    Stems, too)
*10* whole dried pitted dates, cut in 5 pieces
*1/2* cup dried cherries
*1* teaspoon peanut oil to lightly grease the pan

### Instructions
- Preheat oven to 350°
- Add agave nectar, oil, and cinnamon in small bowl and whisk together.
- Then in a large bowl, stir together oats, flour, almonds, sunflower seeds, salt and dried fruit.
- Then add the agave mixture to the oatmeal fruit mixture. Using your hands, work together until mixed well.
- Place in a lightly oiled 8X8 pan and press ingredients down tightly. Moisten your hands with water before pressing into the pan, this keeps the mixture from sticking to your hands.
- Bake at 350 for 25 min.

- Let set for 15 min. on a cooling rack and cut into 12 equal bars.

### Recipe Notes

*Kitchen Tips*:

*I use kitchen scissors to cut the dried fruit into pieces, it is easier than trying to use a knife.*

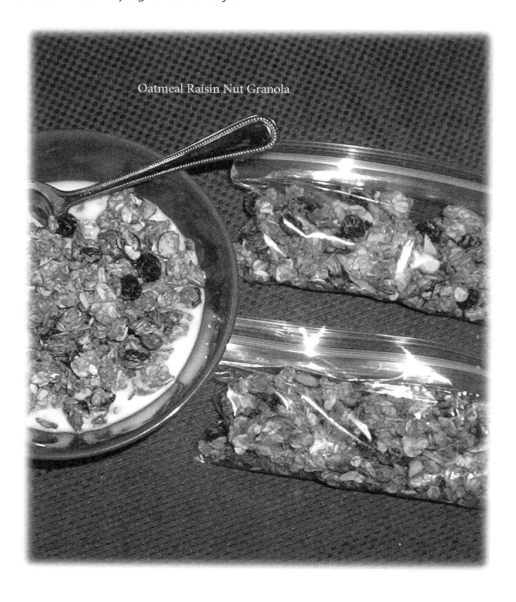

Oatmeal Raisin Nut Granola

# Oatmeal Raisin Nut Granola

*1/2* cup raw agave nectar
2 tablespoons peanut oil
1 teaspoon cinnamon
1 ½ cups oats (Old Fashioned), uncooked
*1/2* cup whole-grain wheat flour
*1/2* cup sliced almonds
*1/4* teaspoon salt
*1/2* cup raisins
1 teaspoon peanut oil to lightly grease baking sheet

## Instructions
- Preheat oven to 350°
- Stir together agave, peanut oil and cinnamon in a small bowl.
- Stir together oats, flour, sliced almonds, and salt in a large bowl.
- Add agave mixture to oatmeal mixture, stirring until combined.
- Spread oat mixture onto a lightly greased baking sheet.
- Bake at 350 for 20 minutes, stirring every 5 minutes
- Let cool and store in an airtight container, will keep up to 5 days

## Recipe Notes
*This makes an excellent breakfast cereal. Add a sliced banana or a handful of berries.*

Serves: 6.

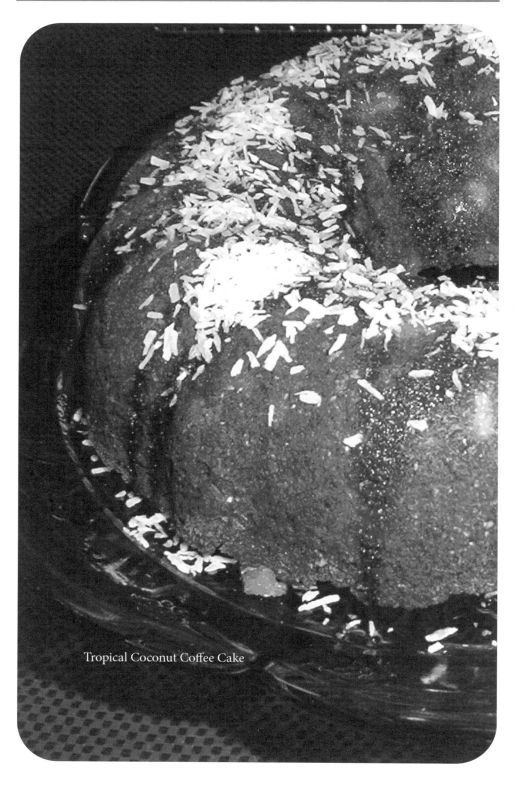

Tropical Coconut Coffee Cake

# Tropical Coconut Coffee Cake

*1* cup raw agave nectar
*1/2* cup coconut oil (organic extra-virgin cold pressed)
2 cups whole-grain wheat flour
*1* teaspoons baking soda
2 teaspoons cinnamon
*1* cup ripe bananas, mashed
*1* 8 oz. can crushed pineapple, drained
*1* teaspoon lemon juice
*1* cup walnuts
*1/2* cup unsweetened coconut flakes
*1* tablespoon of coconut oil (organic extra-virgin cold pressed)
   to lightly oil the pan
For garnishment:
*1/8* cup raw agave nectar
*1* tablespoon shredded coconut

## *Instructions*

- Preheat oven to 350°
- Put a tablespoon of coconut oil in your bundt pan...use a paper towel to coat the oil on all the sides. Add some flour to the pan and toss it around until the bundt pan is lightly floured.
- Combine mashed bananas and well- drained pineapple in a small bowl add lemon juice, set aside.
- In a separate bowl, combine flour, soda, cinnamon and 1/2 cup of coconut flakes, mix well.
- In a large bowl, mix agave nectar and coconut oil. If the coconut oil is solid, melt in the microwave before mixing with the agave nectar.

- Alternatively add banana mixture and flour mixture to the agave mixture until all is mixed together.
- Fold in 1 cup of chopped walnuts.
- Pour into the bundt pan and bake at 350° for 25-30 min or until a toothpick comes out clean.
- Let sit on a cooling rack for 30-45 min. Then loosen the sides with a knife before turning over on a serving plate.
- Drizzle the top with agave nectar and sprinkle with shredded  coconut flakes

### Recipe Notes

*Test kitchens have noted a 25° to 50° temperature difference in ovens. Because of this temperature difference, it will be important for you to check your cake 5 to 10 min before the directions indicate it is done. Insert a toothpick in the center of the loaf, if it comes out clean the cake is done.*

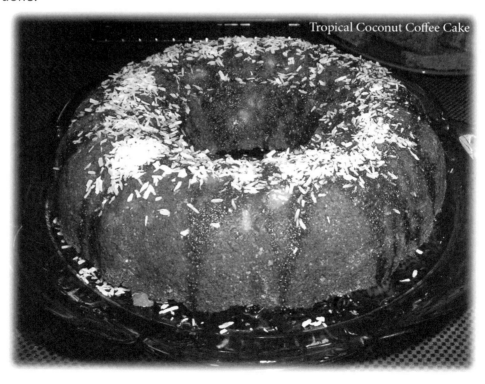

Tropical Coconut Coffee Cake

# Snacks

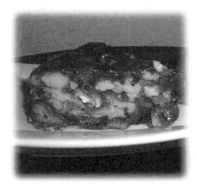
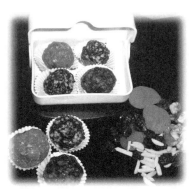

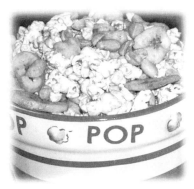

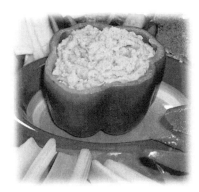
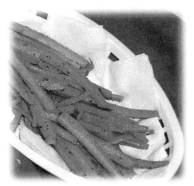

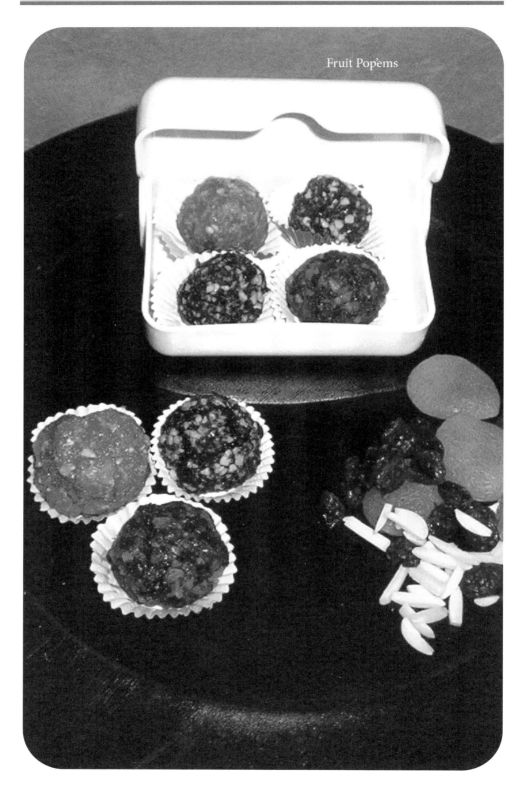

Fruit Pop'ems

# Apricot Fruit Pop'ems

*2* cups dried apricots
*1* cup pecans
*1* tablespoon orange juice

### Instructions

- Dump all of the above ingredients in a food processor and pulse for about 30 seconds.
- Then make into small balls about the size of a quarter
- Refrigerate in tight container

### Recipe Notes

These are great to put in baggies and take as a quick pick- me up snack. As pictured, these fit perfectly in a travel soap dish.

# Fig Fruit Pop'ems

*1* cup dried figs
*1* cup golden seedless raisin
*1* cup walnuts
*1* tablespoon orange juice

### Instructions

- Dump all of the above ingredients in a food processor and pulse for about 30 seconds.
- Then make into small balls about the size of a quarter
- Refrigerate in tight container

### Recipe Notes

*These are great to put in baggies and take as a quick pick- me up snack. As pictured, these fit perfectly in a travel soap dish.*

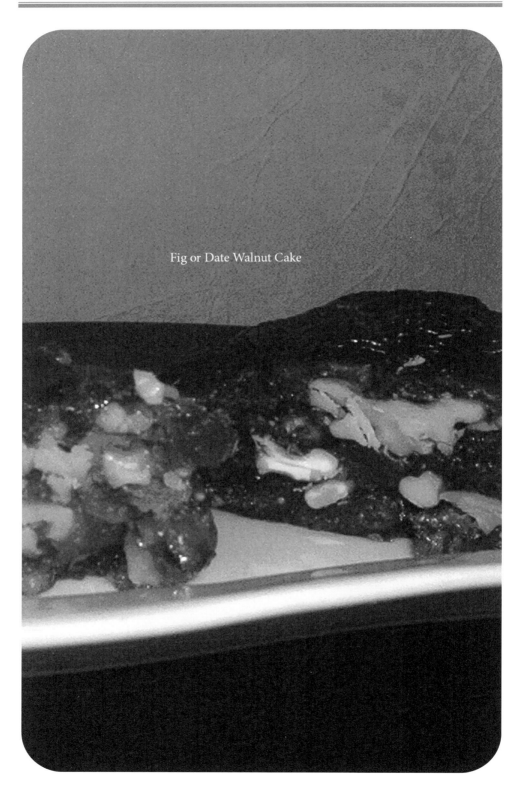

Fig or Date Walnut Cake

# Fig or Date Walnut Cake

2  10 oz. bags of dried gooey figs or *2* -10 oz bags of gooey
  dates ( no pits)
*2* cups walnut halves

**Instructions**
- You will need a 6" diameter mini cake pan or mini cheesecake pan.
- Place cellophane on the inside of the pan you are using, making sure you have plenty to overlap the top when you are done.
- Using a pair of scissors, cut open one side of the fruit
- In the first layer, line the bottom with the fruit gooey side up
- Then cover with walnut halves, just enough to make one layer, with the palm of your hand press down and mash the walnuts in to the figs
- Then repeat the process with the second layer of figs and then the walnuts, press once again...
- To finish the top, place the sticky side down for the top layer. Fold the cellophane over the top and press all around many times.
- To remove from the pan,  pull up on the cellophane
- Put on a cutting board and cut small pieces. Wrap individually in cellophane for a quick and healthy snack.

Does not need refrigeration...great for trips and hunger buster's or an impressive dessert.

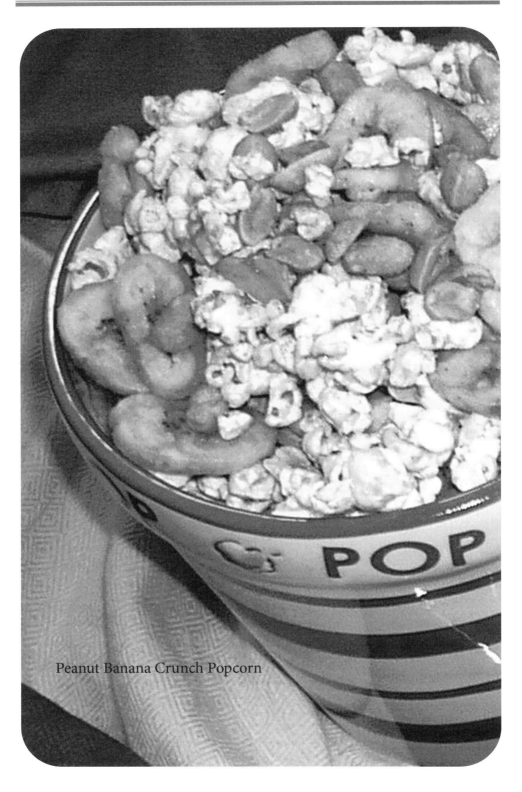

Peanut Banana Crunch Popcorn

# Peanut Banana Crunch Popcorn

*5* quarts popcorn, (about 20 cups popped popcorn)
*2* cups dried banana chips
*1/2* cup natural peanut butter
*2* tablespoons peanut oil
*2* teaspoons Braggs (Alternative to Soy Sauce)
*1/4* teaspoon garlic powder
*1/4* teaspoon cayenne pepper
*1* cup peanuts

### Instructions

- Preheat oven to 275°
- In a large pan, combine popped popcorn, banana chips and peanuts.
- In a small saucepan, combine peanut butter, oil, Braggs, garlic powder, cayenne pepper and stir over medium heat until melted. Pour mixture over the popcorn and toss.
- Spread popcorn on a cookie sheet and bake in oven for 15 minutes. Toss several times.

Serves: 6.

# Pineapple Coconut Granola

*1* cup raw agave nectar
*2* tablespoons coconut oil (organic extra-virgin cold pressed)
*1* teaspoon cinnamon
*1 1/2* cups oats (Old Fashioned), uncooked
*1/2* cup whole-grain wheat flour
*1* teaspoon salt
*2/3* cup sunflower seed
*1/2* cup walnuts, chopped
*2/3* cup orange juice
*1* cup dried pineapple, cut into bits
*10* whole dried apricots, cut into bits
*10* whole dried plums, cut into bits
*2* cups coconut flakes, unsweetened

## Instructions
- Preheat oven to 250°
- In a small bowl, mix raw agave nectar, coconut oil and cinnamon set aside.
- In a large bowl mix the remaining ingredients, add raw agave nectar mixture to the oatmeal fruit mixture
- Using your hands work together
- When mixed crumble onto a cookie sheet. Bake at 250° for 1 hour

## Recipe Notes
*Make a big batch of granola and put serving sizes in ziploc baggies, then freeze to keep fresh.*

Serves: 6.

# Trail Mix

*1* cup oats (Old Fashioned)
*1* cup whole grain, whole wheat flour
*1* cup dried cranberries
*1* cup cashew nuts, unsalted
*1/2* cup cherries, dried
*1/2* cup walnuts
*1/2* cup sunflower seed
*1/2* cup almond slices
*1/2* cup flax seeds
*1/2* cup pepitas (pumpkin seed kernels)
*1* teaspoon salt
*1* cup raw agave nectar
*1/2* cup peanut oil
*1/4* cup pure natural maple syrup

### Instructions

- Preheat oven to 375°
- In a large bowl, mix oats, flour, salt, cranberries, cherries, walnuts, sunflower seeds, almond slices, flax seeds and toss.
- In a small bowl, combine agave nectar, peanut oil and maple syrup mix until well blended.
- Add agave mixture to the dry mixture and mix well
- Crumble the trail mix on a cookie sheet and bake at 375° for 10-12min.

### Recipe Notes

*This is a great snack or breakfast on the go. All the seeds and nuts provide a great source of protein.*

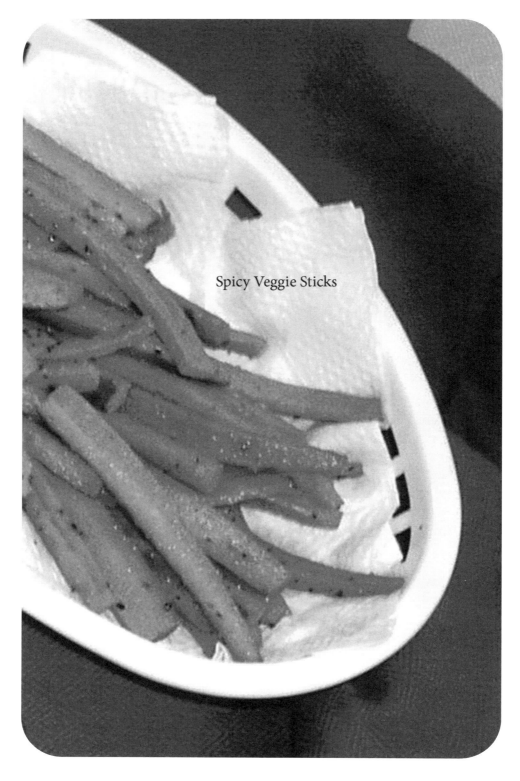

Spicy Veggie Sticks

# Spicy Veggie Sticks

Spicy House Seasoning to taste (recipe follows)
2 tablespoons olive oil
6 carrots, washed
4 potatoes, washed

## *Instructions*

- Preheat the oven to 450°
- Clean and peel the above vegetables. Cut them into thick sticks resembling fries.
- Toss them in the olive oil until coated evenly.
- Place them in a single layer on a cookie sheet and bake them on the top rack for 20 min (or until crispy) turning them every 5 min.
- While hot sprinkle with House Spicy Seasoning mix (to taste)   (recipe follows)

### Spicy House Seasoning

3/4 teaspoon celery seed
3/4 teaspoon paprika
1/2 teaspoon cayenne pepper
1 tablespoon ground mustard seed
1 tablespoon onion powder
2 tablespoons garlic powder
2 tablespoons salt
2 tablespoons pepper

## *Instructions*

Combine all the spices together in a jar. Use leftovers to spice things up!

# Roasted Garlic Hummus

*1* 15 oz. can garbanzo bean, rinsed & drained
*2* tablespoons tahini
*2* tablespoons olive oil
*1/4* cup lemon juice
*20* whole garlic cloves, roasted
*1* teaspoon salt
*1/4* cup water

### Instructions

Roasted Garlic:

- Preheat oven to 400°
- You will need about 2 heads of garlic...there is about 10 cloves per head. Peel the outside skin off the garlic head.
- Then cut about 1/4" off the top of each head.
- Drizzle about 1 teaspoon of olive oil over the head of garlic and loosely wrap it in aluminum foil.
- Bake in the oven for 20min. Garlic should easily slip out of its casing.

Hummus:

- Place all the ingredients in a food processor and blend on high for 2-3 min.

### Recipe Notes

I love to spread this on whole grain tortillas then add thinly (like paper thin) zucchini, squash and lettuce on the hummus. Then I gently roll it up. Makes great pin wheels  or a wrap!

# Roasted Red Pepper Hummus

*1* 15 oz. can garbanzo bean, rinsed & drained
*1* whole red bell pepper, roasted
*1* tablespoon tahini
*1* tablespoon olive oil
*1/4* cup lemon juice
*6* whole garlic cloves, roasted
*1* tablespoon tomato paste
*1* teaspoon salt
*1/4* cup water

### Instructions
Roasted Bell Pepper and Garlic:
- Preheat the oven to 400°
- Cut the red bell pepper in half length wise. Clean out all the seeds.
- Place on a cookie sheet skin up.
- Now prepare the garlic
- Peel the outer skin off the garlic head.
- Then cut 1/4" off the top and drizzle with 1 teaspoon of olive oil.
- Loosely wrap the garlic head in aluminum foil.
- Place on the same cookie sheet as the bell pepper
- Bake for about 20 min. Remove from the oven and place the bell pepper in a zip loc bag for 5 min.
- After the pepper has set, peel the skin off. The garlic cloves should easily slip out.

Hummus:
Place all the ingredients in a food processor and blend on high for 2-3 min.

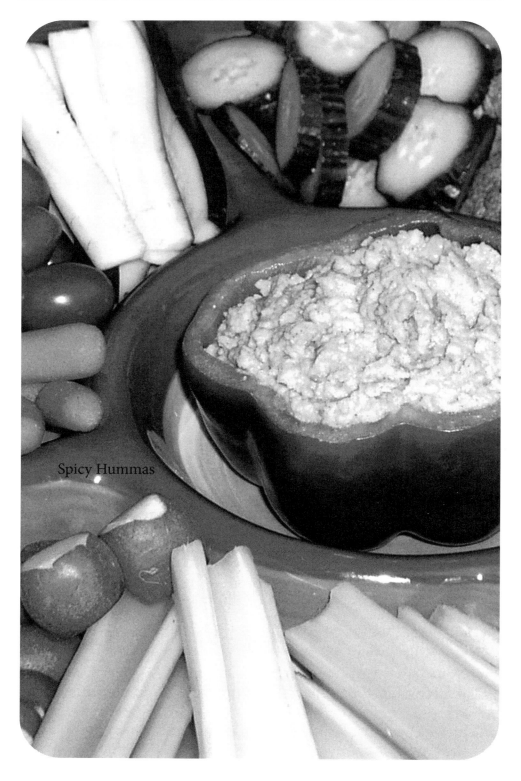

Spicy Hummas

# Spicy Hummus

*1* can chickpeas, drained and rinsed
*1/4* cup sesame seed
*1* tablespoon olive oil
*1* tablespoon minced garlic
*1* teaspoon cumin
*1* teaspoon coriander
*1/2* teaspoon red pepper
*1/2* teaspoon salt
*1* whole lemon, juiced

### Instructions

- In a food processor, puree sesame seeds and olive oil.
- Add chickpeas, minced garlic, cumin, coriander, red pepper, salt and lemon juice.
- Blend until smooth.

Serve with vegetables or spread on a whole wheat tortilla. Makes a meal by adding tomatoes, onions and lettuce to your whole wheat tortilla

# Main Dishes, Soups and Salads

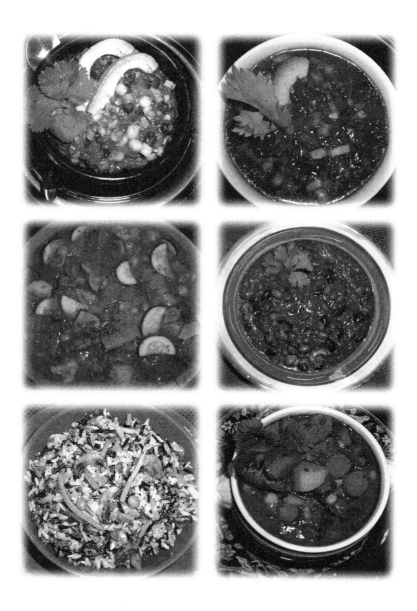

# Cinnamon-Honey Acorn Squash

*1* medium acorn squash, cut in half (stem to end)
*2* tablespoons olive oil, 1 tablespoon for each half
*2* tablespoons cinnamon, 1 tablespoon for each half
*2* tablespoons raw agave nectar, 1 tablespoon for each half
*1* pinch salt, to taste
*1/4* cup water

## *Instructions*
- Cut the acorn in half from the pointy end to the stem and clean out the seeds.
- Place both halves in a glass bread pan and add 1/4 cup of water in the bottom.
- Put olive oil in coating the inside of each squash, shake on cinnamon and salt.
- Cover with a plastic wrap, that is microwave safe
- cook in the microwave for 10 min's
- Let set for 3 minutes, be careful taking off the plastic wrap it will be steamy.
- Add more raw agave nectar or cinnamon to taste

# Orange Cranberry Couscous

*1* cup whole wheat couscous
*1 1/2* cups orange juice
*1* tablespoon olive oil
*1/2* cup dried cranberries
*1/3* cup parsley, chopped
*1* cup toasted slivered almonds
*1* teaspoon pepper
*1* teaspoon salt

### Instructions

- In a sauce pan, bring orange juice and olive oil to a boil, add couscous and remove from heat
- Stir and cover for 5 min
- Then, fluff with a fork.
- Add remaining ingredients...may be served warm or as a cold salad.

Very yummy! This is one of my favorite recipes! I suggest doubling the recipe, just to have some for another day.

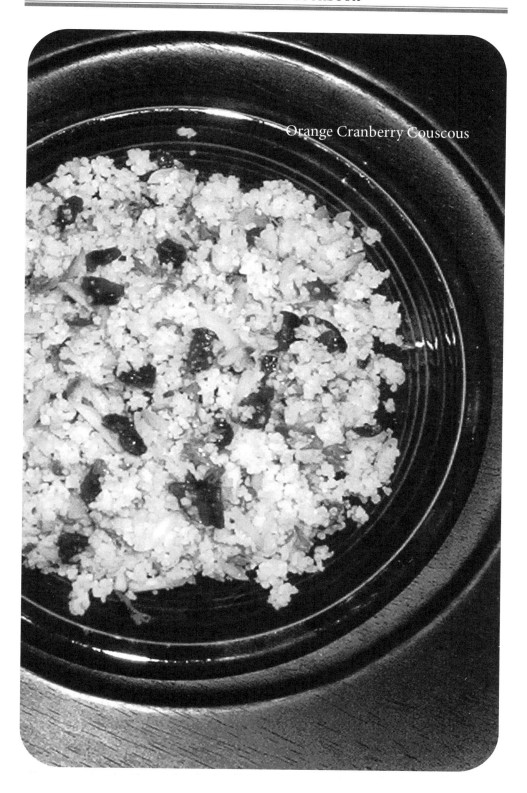

Orange Cranberry Couscous

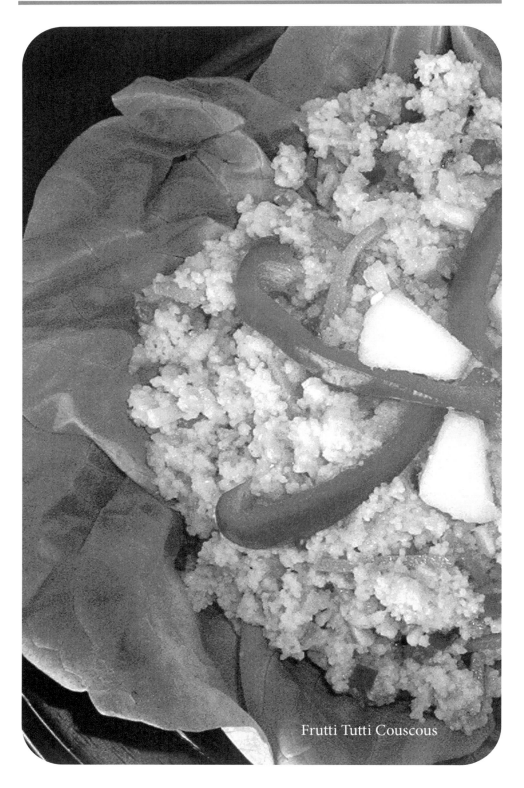

Frutti Tutti Couscous

# FRUTTI TUTTI COUSCOUS

*1 1/4* cups orange juice

*1* cup water

*1* teaspoon salt

*1* teaspoon pepper

*1* tablespoon olive oil

*1 1/2* cups whole wheat couscous (1- 7.6oz. box whole grain
   wheat couscous)

*1/2* cup shredded carrot

*1/2* cup frozen pineapple chunks (approximately 8 pieces)
   chopped w/Vidalia Chopper

*1/2* cup frozen mango chunks (approximately 8 pieces)
   chopped w/Vidalia Chopper

*1* cup toasted pine nuts

*1* half jalapeno pepper seeded, chopped w/Vidalia Chopper
   fine insert

*1* half red bell pepper, chopped w/Vidalia Chopper fine insert

*1/4* purple onion, chopped w/Vidalia Chopper fine insert

*1* zest of one lime

## *Instructions*

- Put orange juice, water, salt, pepper and olive oil in a microwaveable glass dish and bring to a boil in the microwave (takes about 6 min).
- Then add couscous and cover for 5 min.
- In the meantime, in a large bowl combine all the other ingredients.
- After couscous has set for 5 min's fluff with fork and add to the large bowl and stir to mix. Serve cold.

If you like cilantro, chop it and garnish. This is a great taste combination. This dish makes a wonderful take to work lunch!

# Couscous

*2* stalks celery, finely chopped
*1* small white onion, finely chopped
*8* ounces mushrooms, finely chopped
*2* cloves garlic, finely chopped
*3* tablespoons olive oil
*1* cup Whole Wheat Couscous
*1* teaspoon rosemary, ground
*1* teaspoon paprika, ground
*1* teaspoon turmeric, ground
*1* teaspoon cinnamon, ground
*1* teaspoon chili powder
*1* cup vegetable broth, can substitute with water
*1* teaspoon coriander, ground

### Instructions

- In a large bowl, add the couscous and spices
- Pour 1 cup of boiling hot vegetable broth or water and cover with a plate
- In a sauté pan, add the olive oil and all vegetables
- Cook until mushrooms are tender, this usually takes just a few minutes.
- Remove lid from couscous bowl and gently fluff with a fork
- Add sautéed vegetables, salt and pepper to taste

### Recipe Notes

*Use the finer chop insert on the Vidalia Chop Wizard to finely chop the vegetables. To learn more about the Vidalia chopper see page 41*

# Pecan Pear Salad

*1* 15 oz bag of mixed salad greens
*2* 15 oz. can pears halves, canned, No sugar added
*1/2* cup toasted pecans
*1/2* cup dried cranberries

Sweet Maple Salad Dressing (recipe on following page)

## Instructions

- Divide the mixed greens into desired serving sizes.
- Slice the pears into nice sized wedges and distribute evenly over the salads.
- Heat the toasted pecans in the microwave... it should only take a min or two.
- Evenly distribute the pecans and cranberries on the salad.
- Make the Sweet Maple Salad Dressing described below and drizzle over the salad. Enjoy!

## Recipe Notes

*Fresh Pears are better! Substitute one large pear for each can.*
*To toast the pecans, pre heat the oven to 350°.*
*Spread the nuts on an ungreased shallow pan and bake for 10 min. Stir occasionally.*

# Sweet Maple Salad Dressing

*1/4* cup maple syrup
*2* tablespoons lemon juice
*1* teaspoon dry mustard
*1/4* teaspoon salt
*1/4* teaspoon pepper
*1/4* cup olive oil

### Instructions
Add all the ingredients to a small bowl and mix thoroughly

# Peanut Pesto Macaroni Salad

*4* cups whole grain macaroni noodles (No Egg), cooked
*2* cups carrots, shredded
*2* cups frozen peas
*1* cup cilantro leaves
*1 ½ inches* whole ginger root, peeled
*3/4* cup green onion, chopped
*1/4* cup all natural peanut butter
*1/4* cup peanuts, for topping
*1/4* cup olive oil
*2* teaspoons lemon juice
*1* teaspoon salt
*1/2* teaspoon pepper

## Instructions

- Cook macaroni according to directions, adding carrots and peas during the last 2 min's of cooking RESERVE 1/2 CUP OF COOKING WATER then DRAIN
- Put drained cooked pasta in a bowl
- Meanwhile, in the food processor, puree' garlic, cilantro, ginger, green onions, olive oil, peanut butter, lemon juice, salt and pepper until smooth.
- Then add cooking water (if you forget the pasta water ..just add hot water
- Toss macaroni with cilantro mixture. Sprinkle peanuts over the top. Salt and pepper to taste.

May be served hot or at room temp.

## Recipe Notes

**Family Friendly**: *After portions have been removed for those on the Daniel's Fast, add cooked chicken. I like to pick up an*

*already cooked rotisserie chicken from my local grocery store. Simply take the chicken off the bones and wha-la!*
**Short cuts**: *Use the pre-shredded carrots in the produce aisle. Fresh lemon juice can be found in the freezer section.*

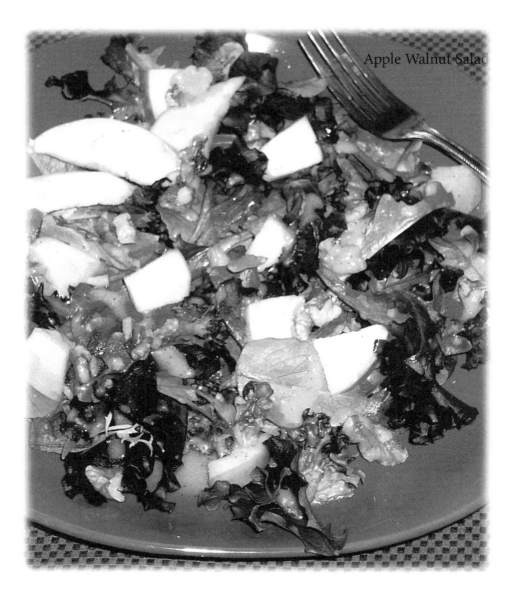

Apple Walnut Salad

# Apple Walnut Salad

*1* 15 oz bag of mixed salad greens
*1* medium apple
*1/2* cup toasted walnuts
Apple Walnut Salad Dressing (recipe on following page)

## Instructions

- Make the Apple Walnut Salad Dressing as described below.
- Toast walnuts, core the apple and cut into bite sized pieces. In a large bowl, toss the greens, apple pieces, toasted walnuts and salad dressing.

## Recipe Notes

*To toast the walnuts, preheat the oven to 350°.*
*Spread the nuts on an ungreased shallow pan and bake for 10 min. Stir occasionally.*
**Family Friendly Version**: *For family members that are not on the Daniel's Fast, 1/2 cup of Gorgonzola cheese can be added.*

# Apple Walnut Salad Dressing

*1/3* cup olive oil
*1/2* teaspoon walnut oil
*1* tablespoon lemon juice
*3* tablespoons apple juice, frozen
*1* package stevia
*1* teaspoon dry mustard
*1* tablespoon minced garlic, jar ok
*1/4* teaspoon salt
*1/8* teaspoon ground cloves

### Instructions

- Place all ingredients in a food processor and mix on high for 1 minutes

### Recipe Notes

The stevia package is an individual sized package sold under the name Sweet Leaf. I have purchased a box of 100 count packets from Wal-Mart. The individual sized packet contains 1/4 teaspoon of stevia.

# Southwest Pasta Sa

*1* 15 oz. can black bean, rinsed
*1* 11 oz. can corn, drained
*1* 8 oz. box whole wheat spiral pasta
*1* whole red bell pepper, chopped fine
*1* medium white onion, chopped fine
*1* whole jalapeno pepper, seeded & chopped fine
*2* medium tomatoes, chopped fine
*1* whole lime, zest
Cilantro Dressing (recipe on following page)

## Instructions
- Rinse the black beans and place in a large bowl
- Add drained corn and cooked spiral pasta
- Toss in the zest of one lime
- Use the fine insert of the Vidalia Chopper to chop the remaining ingredients and add them to the bowl.
- Prepare the Cilantro Dressing and stir into the medley of vegetables. Serve at room temperature.

## Recipe Notes
*When purchasing the whole wheat spiral pasta, make sure there isn't any egg in the ingredients.*

# Cilantro Dressing

*1* bunch cilantro leaves
*2* teaspoons minced garlic, jar ok
*2* teaspoons salt
*1* teaspoon pepper
*1* teaspoon cumin
*1/3* cup olive oil
*1* whole lime, juiced

**Instructions**
*Place all the ingredients in a food processor and blend for one minute*

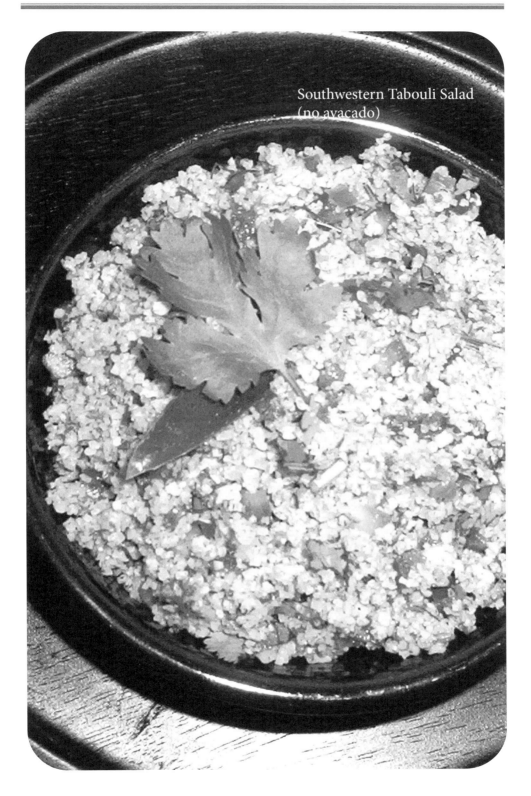

Southwestern Tabouli Salad (no avacado)

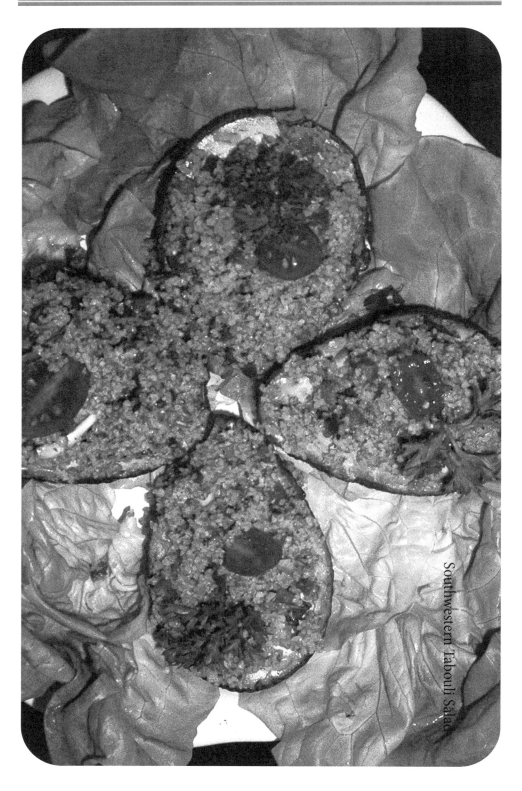

Southwestern Tabouli Salad

# Southwestern Tabouli Salad

*1* 6 oz. box Tabouli Salad made by Fantastic World Foods
*1 ¼* cups water
*2* tablespoons olive oil
*1* large tomato, diced
*1* small jalapeno pepper seeded, diced
*1* half green pepper, diced
*1* bunch cilantro leaves, chopped fine
*1* half purple onion, chopped
*4* whole avocados

## Instructions

- Place tabouli mixture in a salad bowl and add 1 1/4 cups of boiling water and 2 Tbsp of olive oil, stir and cover and put in the refrigerator for 1 hour.
- In the meantime, in a small bowl, add diced tomato, jalapeno, bell pepper and cilantro; mix together.
- When tabouli has cooled...fluff with a fork...add tomato mixture and stir until blended
- Cut avocados in half and mound mixture on top...makes 8 halves

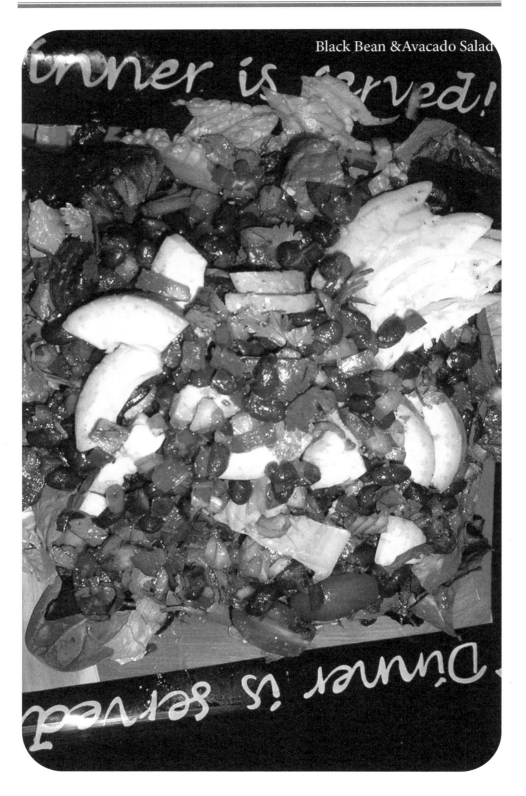

Black Bean &Avacado Salad

# Black Bean and A\

*1* 15 oz. can black bean, drained and r
*1* cup red bell pepper, chopped w/Vida
*1/2* cup red onion, chopped w/Vidalia fi
*1* whole jalapeno pepper seeded, choppe
*1* whole avocado, diced
*1/4* cup chopped fresh cilantro
*4* tablespoons lime juice
*2* tablespoons olive oil
*1/2* teaspoon garlic powder
*1/4* teaspoon pepper
*1/2* teaspoon salt
*6* cups mixed greens

## *Instructions*

- Place the first six ingredients in a bowl.
- Then in a separate bowl whisk together the lime juice, olive oil and seasonings.
- Pour the mixture over the black bean mixture. Mound mixture over greens. May add more salt or lime juice to taste

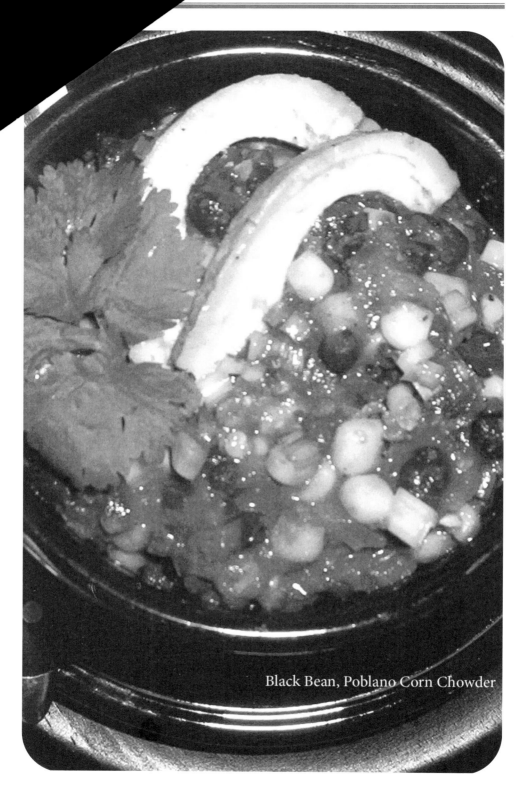

Black Bean, Poblano Corn Chowder

# Black Bean, Poblano Corn Chowder

*2* whole poblano peppers (or Anaheim peppers)
*2* 15 oz. can black beans, drained
*2* tablespoons olive oil
*1* tablespoon chopped garlic, jar ok
*1* tablespoon ground cumin
*1* teaspoon pepper
*1* teaspoon salt
*2* tablespoons dried parsley
*2* 14.5 oz. can diced tomatoes
*2* cups frozen corn
*1* large onion, chopped with Vidalia fine insert, about 2 cups

## *Instructions*

- Place the poblano peppers on the grill and char them on all sides
- Place  peppers in a bowl and cover tightly with wrap after about 5 minutes, remove the skin, stem and seeds
- Drop in food processor and blend. This adds great flavor to the soup...however, if time does not allow you to do this..omit peppers it will still be delicious.
- In a large pot, put the olive oil, onions, garlic and sauté for about 5 minutes
- Add the can of tomatoes, juice and all, along with the black beans, corn, poblano peppers and all the seasonings.
- Cover with lid and simmer for 20 minutes. Enjoy!

Serves: 6.

# Split Pea Soup

*1* 16oz.package dried split peas
*8* cups water
*2* cups frozen crinkle cut carrots (sliced)
*3* medium potatoes, chopped w/Vidalia chopper coarse insert
*2* cups onion, chopped with Vidalia fine insert
*2* tablespoons minced garlic, jar ok
*2* teaspoons salt
*1* teaspoon pepper

## Instructions

- Put all the ingredients in a big pot and bring to a boil.
- Reduce heat and simmer with the pot lid ajar for 45 min.

## Recipe Notes

*Goes well with homemade whole-wheat crackers...*
*See recipe in yeast-free bread section*

Serves: 6.

# Potato Soup- Daniel Style

*1* 16 oz. package frozen butter beans
*5* medium potatoes, cut in 1/2" chunks
*1* quart vegetable broth, 32 oz carton
*2* large onion, chopped with Vidalia fine insert, about 4 cups
*1* cup frozen corn
*1* cup frozen peas
*2* teaspoons minced garlic, jar ok
*1* cup frozen crinkle cut carrots
*1* package 8 oz package of sliced white mushrooms
*1* teaspoon salt
*1* teaspoon pepper
*1* teaspoon celery salt

*Instructions*

- In a large pot, add beans, potatoes, carrots and veggie stock
- Bring to a boil and then simmer with lid on for 10 minutes
- In the mean time, in a sauté pan, place 3 Tbsp of olive oil and add onions, mushrooms and garlic...stir for about 3 minutes
- Add the sautéed mixture to the large pot. Add all remain ingredients bring to a boil and simmer for about 10 to 15 minutes or until potatoes are tender

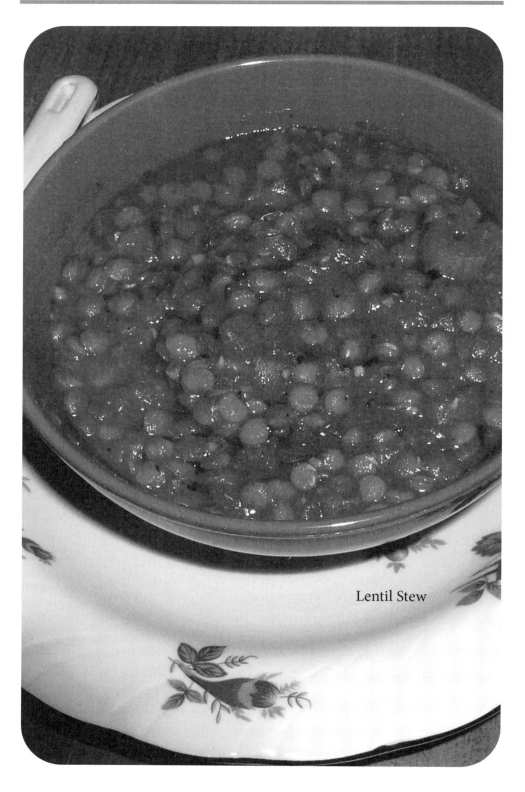

Lentil Stew

# Lentil Stew

*2* tablespoons olive oil
*1* large chopped yellow onion, about 1 cup
*2* tablespoons minced garlic
*1* cup carrot, sliced
*1/2* cup celery, chopped
*5* whole sun-dried tomatoes in olive oil, cut in pieces
*1* 6 oz. can tomato paste
*2* 32 oz. cartons vegetable broth
*2* cups lentils, about 1 pound
*1* 14.5 oz. can diced tomatoes
*1* teaspoon dried oregano
*1/2* tablespoon dried basil
*2* teaspoons salt
*1* teaspoon pepper

## Instructions

- In a large pot, sauté onions in the olive oil until clear
- Add the remaining ingredients and bring to a boil
- Reduce heat and simmer for 1.5 hours or until the carrots are tender

## Recipe Notes

*This makes a thick soup. If you wish for it to be thinner, add 1/2 cup of lentils instead of 1 cup.*

**Family Friendly**: *After removing a portion for those on the Daniel's Fast, add cooked sausage crumbles.*

*Freeze EXTRAS! This works great for quick lunches. I like to freeze this in individual servings. Ziploc makes a container with a screw on lid. It works very well when freezing soups :)*

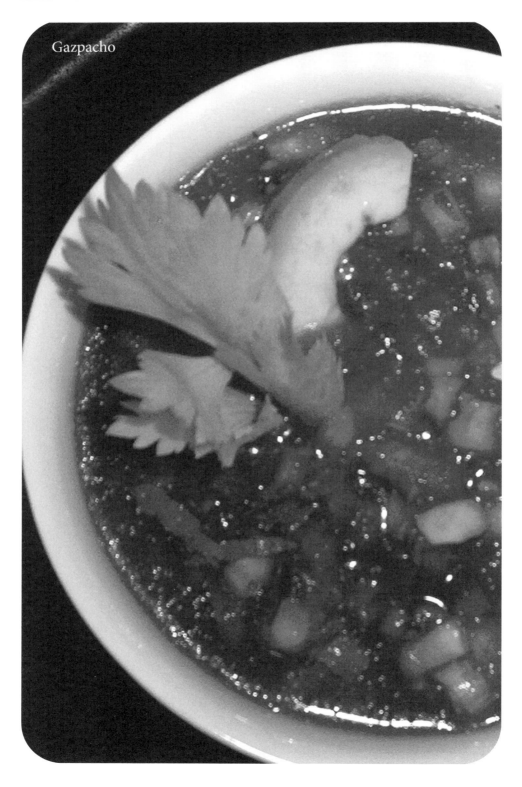

Gazpacho

# Gazpacho -Easy and Refreshing!

*6* large roma tomatoes, chopped w/Vidalia chopper
*1* 12oz. can of tomato juice
*2* tablespoons purple onions, chopped w/Vidalia fine insert
*1* half jalapeno pepper seeded, chopped w/Vidalia fine insert
*1* teaspoon chopped garlic
*1* teaspoon salt
*1* teaspoon pepper
*2* tablespoons lemon juice
*1* cup vegetable broth
*1* half cucumber, chopped w/Vidalia fine insert
*1* half green pepper, chopped w/Vidalia fine insert
*1* stalk of celery chopped w/ Vidalia fine insert
*2* tablespoons cilantro leaves, minced
*4* whole green onions, sliced thin
*1/8* teaspoon red pepper flakes

### Instructions
- Place all ingredients in a bowl and stir to blend
- Serve cold with chopped avocados as garnishment

Serves: 4.

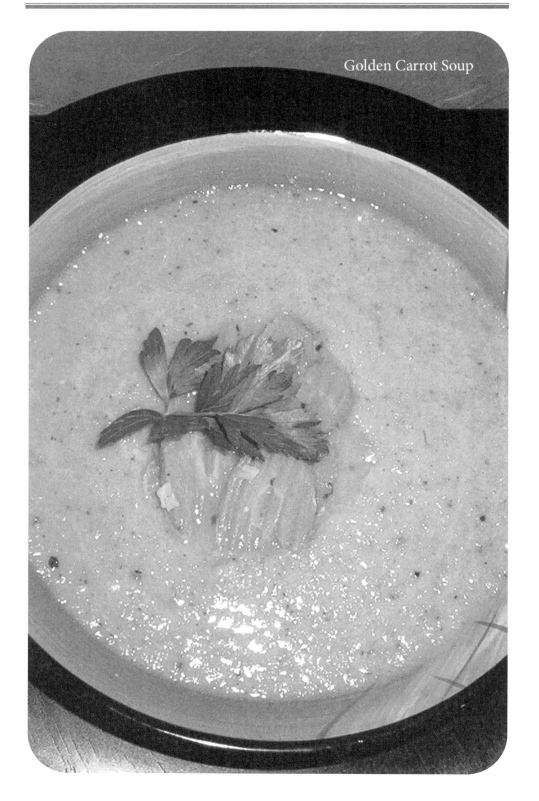

Golden Carrot Soup

# Golden Carrot Soup

2 tablespoons olive oil
1 large onion, chopped with Vidalia fine insert, about 2 cups
3 stalks of celery chopped with Vidalia fine insert, about 1 cup
1 16 oz bag of fresh sliced carrots, about 4 cups
1 quart vegetable broth, 32 oz carton
1 teaspoon poultry seasoning
1 teaspoon dried basil
2 teaspoons chopped garlic, jar ok
1/2 teaspoon pepper
1 teaspoon salt

### Instructions

- In a large pot put olive oil and sauté onion, celery, carrots, garlic and all the seasonings for about 10 minutes.
- Then add the vegetable broth.
- Cover and simmer for about 25 min or until carrots are tender
- With a hand held blender, cream the soup. (If you do not have an hand held blender, spoon into a regular blender. Blend half at a time..be careful this is hot stuff.)

Serves: 6.

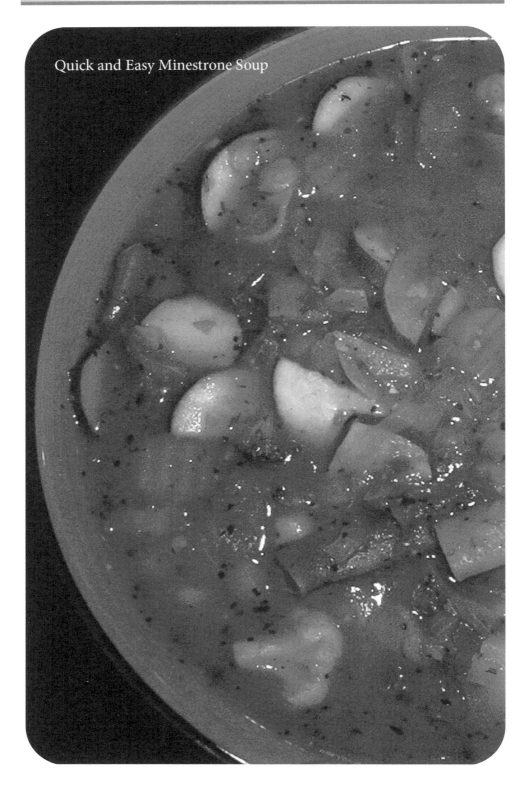

Quick and Easy Minestrone Soup

# Quick and Easy Minestrone Soup

*2* tablespoons olive oil
*2* medium onions, chopped w/Vidalia fine insert
*2* teaspoons chopped garlic
*2* 14.5 oz. can stewed tomatoes w/Italian seasonings
*1* tablespoon tomato paste
*1/2* cup uncooked whole wheat small pasta
*1* 14.5 oz. can garbanzo bean, drained
*1* 16 oz.bag of frozen Italian-style vegetable mix
*1* 14.5 oz. can Italian Cut green beans, drained
*1* teaspoon salt
*1* teaspoon pepper
*1* teaspoon Italian seasoning
*1* teaspoon dried basil

### Instructions

- In a large pot, sauté with olive oil: onions & garlic for a few minutes to sweat
- Add remaining ingredients and bring to a boil
- Stir and cover with lid and simmer for 30 min

This can be put in a crock pot at this point and set on warm for up to 4 hrs. This is a nice meal to come home to after church

Serves: 6.

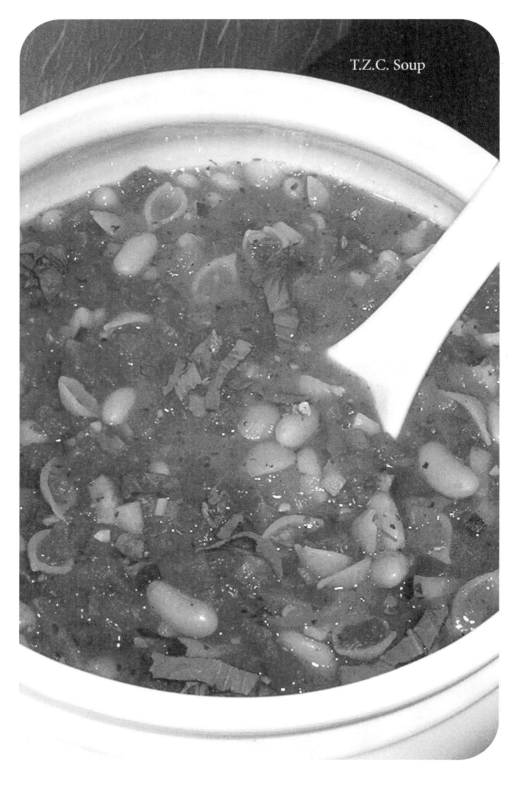

T.Z.C. Soup

# T.Z.C. Soup (Tomato, Zucchini and Conchigliette)

2 tablespoons olive oil
1 medium onion, chopped with Vidalia fine insert, about 1 cup
3 tablespoons chopped garlic, jar ok
1 large zucchini chopped w/Vidalia fine insert, about 1 cup
1/2 cup green pepper, chopped w/Vidalia fine insert
2 15 oz. can diced tomatoes
2 cups vegetable broth
1 teaspoon salt
1 teaspoon pepper
1 teaspoon dried basil
2 teaspoons Italian seasoning
1/4 teaspoon fennel seed
1 tablespoon tomato paste
1 15 oz. can cannellini (white kidney) beans, drained
2/3 cup whole wheat small sea shell pasta (conchigliette), uncooked

## Instructions

- In a large pot place olive oil, onion, garlic, zucchini, green pepper sauté for about 6 minutes
- Then add the tomatoes, vegetable broth, seasonings, tomato paste and beans
- Stir well and bring to a boil
- Then add uncooked pasta and cover and simmer for 15 minutes
- Garnish with fresh basil strips if you have it handy

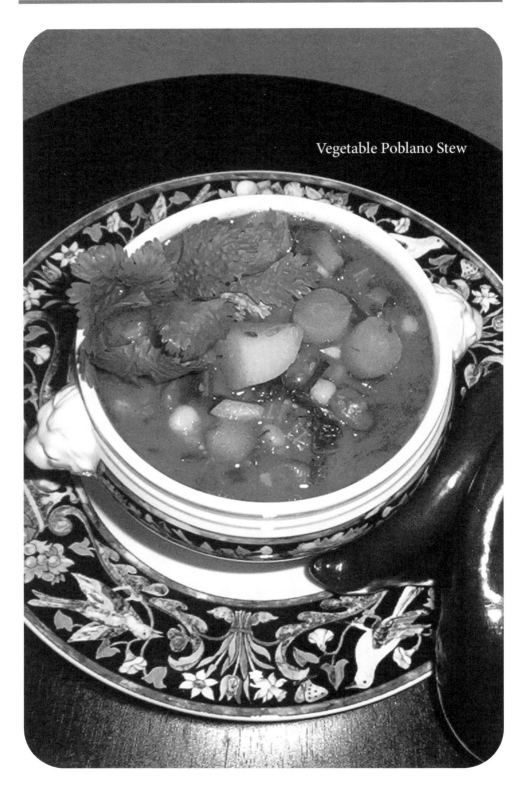

Vegetable Poblano Stew

# Vegetable Poblano Stew

*2* whole poblano peppers (or Anaheim peppers)
*1* tablespoon minced garlic, jar ok
*2* cups onion, chopped with Vidalia fine insert
*1 ½* cups carrots, sliced
*3* stalks of celery chopped with Vidalia fine insert, about ½ cup
*4* whole potatoes, cut in 1" cubes
*2* teaspoons chili powder
*1* teaspoon cumin
*1/2* teaspoon paprika
*2 ½* teaspoons salt
*2* teaspoons pepper
*1* small zucchini chopped w/Vidalia fine insert, about 1 cup
*1 ½* cups frozen corn
*1* 16 oz. can pinto bean, drained
*1* quart vegetable broth, 32 oz carton
*2* cups water
*2* tablespoons olive oil

## *Instructions*
- Remove the stem and seeds from the poblano peppers.
- Then roughly, cut poblano peppers and put them in the food processor. Blend until smooth.
- In a large soup pot, put olive oil on medium high and add garlic, onion, carrots, celery, potatoes, creamed poblano peppers, chili powder, paprika, salt, pepper and cumin.
- Stir for about 15 minutes.
- Stir in zucchini, frozen corn and pinto beans.
- Then pour in the vegetable broth and water. Bring stew to a boil and simmer for about 40 to 45 minutes or until tender.

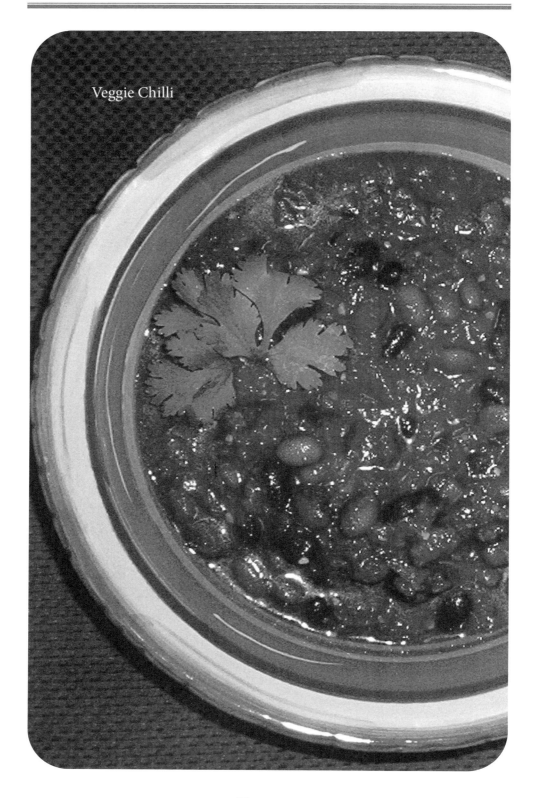

Veggie Chilli

# Veggie Chili (Crock Pot)

*3* tablespoons olive oil
*2* large onion, chopped with Vidalia fine insert, about 4 cups
*1* whole bell pepper, chopped w/Vidalia fine insert
*1* whole jalapeno pepper seeded, chopped w/Vidalia fine insert
*1* tablespoon minced garlic, jar ok
*1* teaspoon salt
*1* teaspoon pepper
*2* teaspoons cumin
*2* tablespoons chili powder
*1* tablespoon tomato paste
*2* 14.5 oz. can diced tomatoes, juice and all
*2* 15 oz. can red kidney beans, juice and all
*1* 15 oz. can pinto bean, juice and all
*1* 15 oz. can pinto bean, drained

## Instructions

- In a large sauté pan, add olive oil, onions, green peppers, jalapeno, garlic and sauté for about 4 minutes.
- Put the sautéed mixture into a crock pot and add remaining ingredients
- Stir and put on high for 2 ½ hours then on warm until ready to eat. Time can be extended by putting on low for 6 hours.

### Recipes Notes

*If you are a Southerner, you may prefer to use only pinto beans*
**Family Friendly Version:** *Fry one pound of hamburger*
*with the following seasoning:*
*salt and pepper*
*2 tsp of Chili powder*
*1/2 tsp of ground cumin*
*Add to the chili after removing Daniel's fast servings*

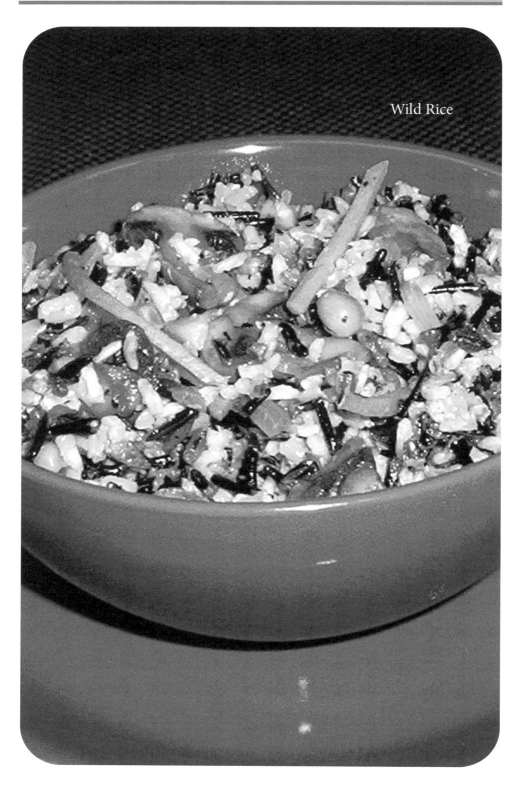

Wild Rice

# Wild Rice

1 ½ cups wild rice (8 oz. package)
1 ½ cups long grain whole brown rice
6 cups water
1 8 oz. package of sliced mushrooms
1 ½ cups onion, chopped with Vidalia fine insert (I large onion)
1/2 cup sliced almonds
2 tablespoons minced garlic, jar ok
1/2 cup carrot, shredded
4 tablespoons olive oil, divided use
2 teaspoons salt
1 teaspoon pepper
1/2 cup frozen green peas

### Instructions

- Bring water, 2 tablespoons of oil and salt to a boil.
- Then add wild rice and boil for 10 minutes uncovered
- Then add long grain brown rice, stir and simmer covered for approximately 55 minutes (water should be absorbed)
- Remove from heat, stir and let it sit for 10 minutes with the lid on
- In a frying pan, add 2 tablespoons of oil, sauté onion, mushrooms, carrots, garlic and almonds until mushrooms are tender (takes about 10-15 minutes)
- Remove the sautéed vegetables from heat and gently toss in frozen peas
- Add vegetable mixture to the mixed rice, stir and serve.

Serves: 8

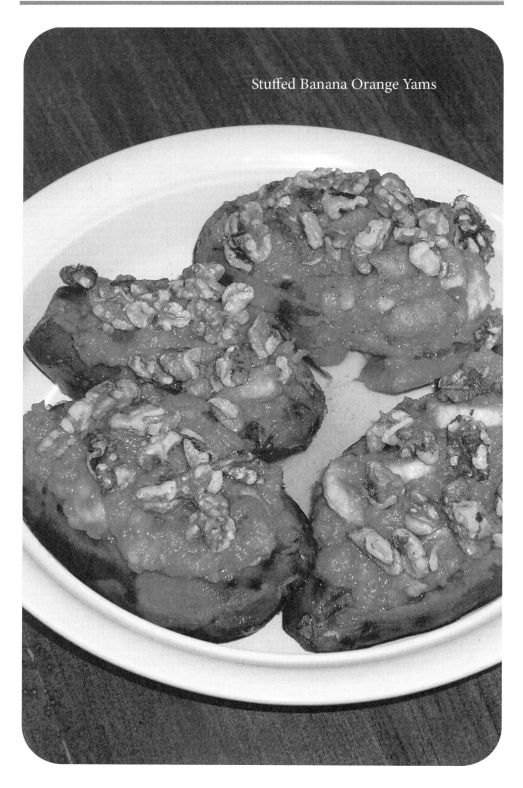

Stuffed Banana Orange Yams

# Stuffed Banana Orange Yams

4 medium yams
1/4 teaspoon pumpkin pie spice
1/2 teaspoon salt
1/3 cup orange juice
1/2 cup walnuts, chopped & roasted
2 whole bananas, ripe
1/8 cup agave nectar

**Instructions**

- Preheat oven to 350°
- Wash sweet potatoes thoroughly and poke holes in the sides. Individually wrap the sweet potatoes in aluminum foil.
- Bake for 45 min to an hour or until done.
- Unwrap the potatoes and gently scoop out the insides.
- In a mixing bowl, add the yam insides, one banana, agave nectar, salt, pumpkin pie spice, orange juice and mash together.
- Then slice the other banana and gently mix into the yam mixture.
- Carefully scoop the yam mixture back into the yam shells and sprinkle with the toasted walnuts.

**Recipe Notes**

*To toast the walnuts, Pre heat the oven to 350°.*
*Spread the nuts on an ungreased shallow pan and bake*
*for 10 min. Stir occasionally.*

Serves: 4.

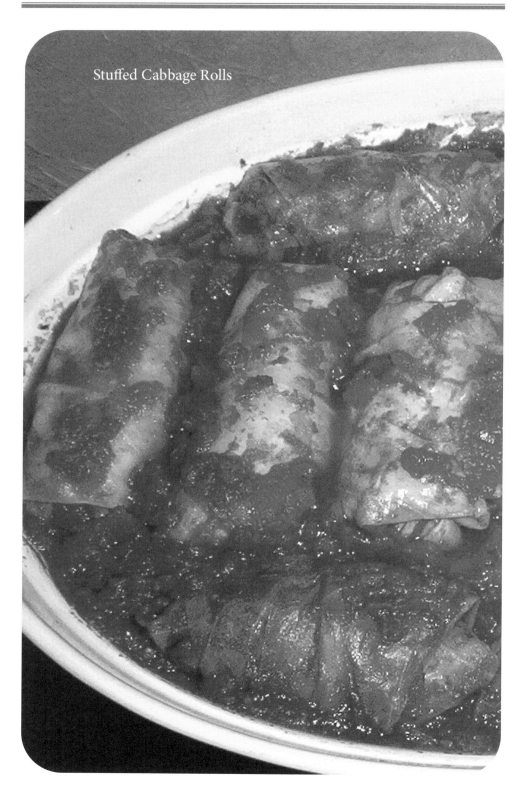

Stuffed Cabbage Rolls

# Stuffed Cabbage Rolls

*1* large head of cabbage, outer leaves removed
*2* tablespoons olive oil
*2* large onions chopped w/ Vidalia coarse insert, about 4 cups
*1* 8 oz package of sliced white mushrooms, chopped
*2* teaspoons chopped garlic, divided use
*2* teaspoons dried parsley
*1/4* teaspoon paprika
*1 ½* cups brown rice, cooked
*1* teaspoon salt
*1/2* teaspoon thyme
*2* 14 oz. cans diced tomatoes
*1* 8 oz. can tomato sauce
*1* 6 oz. can tomato paste
*1/4* cup water

## *Instructions*

- Preheat oven to 350°
- In a large pot, boil the cabbage for about 10 - 15 minutes or until leaves are softened enough to peel away
- Cool and separate leaves.
- While waiting for cabbage to cool, sauté onions in the olive oil for about 6 min
- Remove half of the onions, set aside
- Add mushrooms to the pan along with 1 tsp of garlic, parsley and paprika. Cook for about 4 minutes.
- Pour the sautéed mixture in a bowl with the cooked rice.
- In the now empty pan, add the half of onions that were set aside and add diced tomatoes (juice and all), tomato sauce, tomato paste, water, salt, pepper, garlic and thyme.   Simmer for 15 min.

- Place a heaping tablespoon of rice mixture on each cabbage leaf
- Fold leaf over to enclose rice mixture. Starting at the stem end and roll up.
- Place rolls, seam side down in a dish brushed with olive oil,
- Cover with tomato mixture and bake uncovered for 1 ½ hours at 350°

Serves: 6.

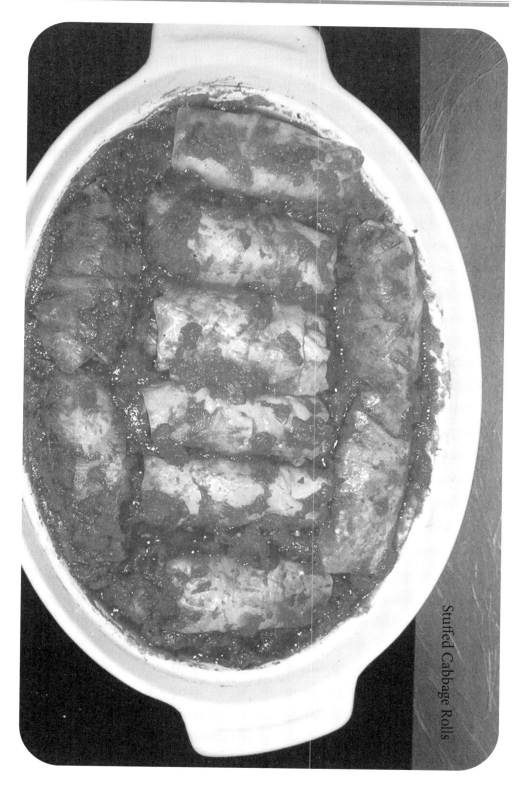

Stuffed Cabbage Rolls

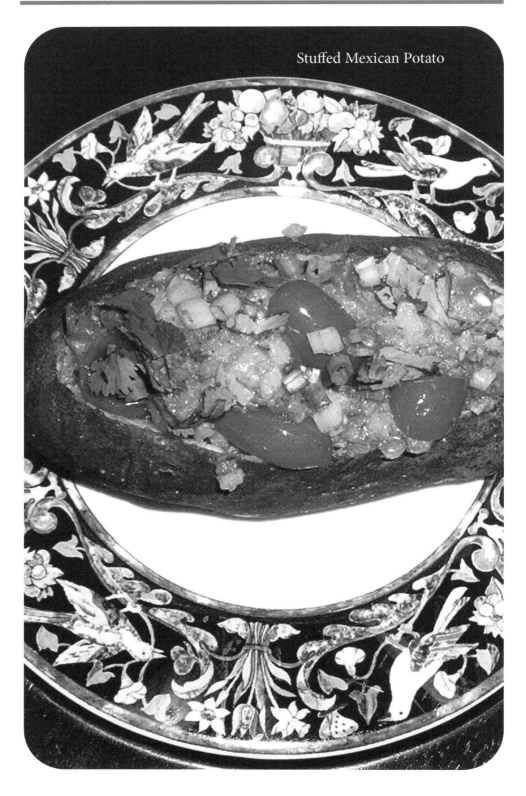

Stuffed Mexican Potato

# Stuffed Mexican Potato

*1* large baking potato
*1/4* cup onion, chopped with Vidalia fine insert
*6* whole grape tomatoes cut in half
*1/4* teaspoon cumin
*1/4* teaspoon chili powder
*6* whole green onions, chopped
*1/4* teaspoon pepper
*1/4* teaspoon salt
*1* tablespoon olive oil
*3* sprigs cilantro leaves
*1* tablespoon Simple Salsa (recipe follows)

### *Instructions*

- Pre heat oven to 425°
- Wash and dry the potato then prick the top several times with a fork.
- Coat the outside of the potato with olive oil and rub salt on the outside
- Place the potato in the center of the oven and bake for approximately 1 hour or until potato is done. Let cool.
- In the meantime, in a small skillet put olive oil, chopped onions and green peppers. Sauté for a few minutes.
- Then add cumin, chili powder, garlic powder, 1 tablespoon of salsa, pepper and salt. Stir for a few minutes and set aside.
- Cut the top off of the potato and carefully remove the inside of the potato... do not scrape to close to the skin
- Mix the potato insides with the sautéed mixture and put back into the potato shell
- Garnish with chopped green onions and cilantro leaves.

# Simple Salsa

*5* whole roma tomatoes, diced
*1/2* whole white onion, diced
*1* whole jalapeno pepper, diced fine
*1/2* cup cilantro leaves, torn
*1* tablespoon chopped garlic, jar ok
*1* tablespoon of lemon juice
*1/2* teaspoon black pepper
*1* teaspoon salt

### Instructions

- Use the Vidalia Chop Wizard coarse insert to dice the Roma tomatoes and onion, place in a large bowl.
- Use the small dice insert of the chop wizard to finely dice the jalapeno, add to the tomatoes and onion.
- Next add, the cilantro leaves, lemon juice, chopped garlic, pepper and salt.
- Stir until mixed well. Makes 3 cups

# Asian Dishes

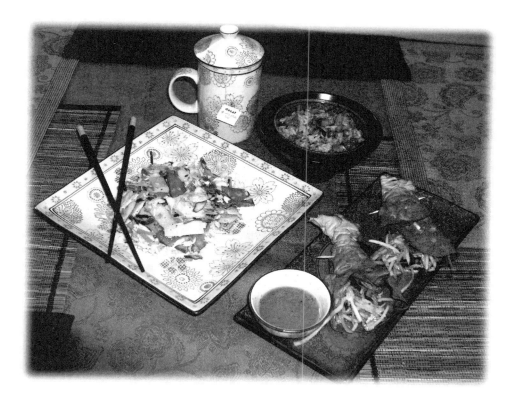

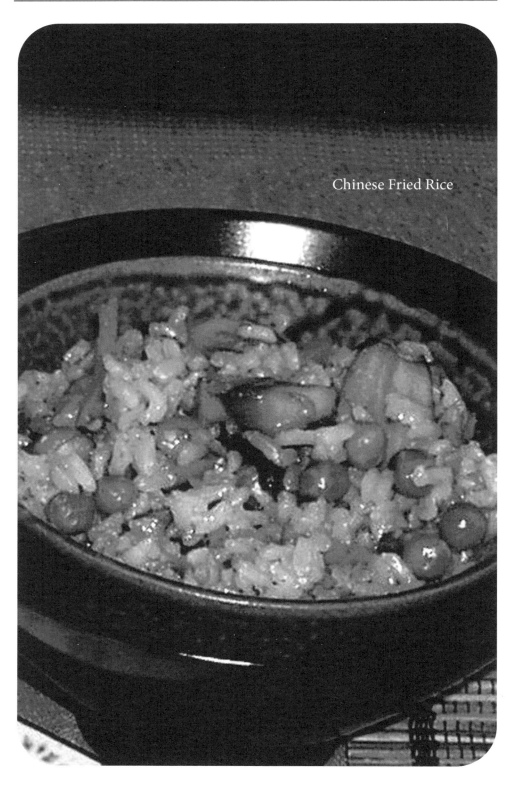

Chinese Fried Rice

# Chinese Fried Rice

*3* tablespoons peanut oil
*1* cup green onion, chopped
*1* 8 oz package sliced fresh mushrooms
*1* cup frozen peas
*1* cup shredded carrot
*4* cups whole grain brown rice, cooked
*1/2* cup dry roasted peanuts
*1/4* cup Braggs (alternative to soy sauce), cooked

## Instructions

- In a Wok heat oil over med-hi heat. Add green onions, mushrooms and carrots.
- Sauté until the mushrooms turn from a light tan to a med brown color
- Stir constantly, add rice then break the rice up and stir into the vegetables.
- Then add the peas, peanuts and Braggs.
- Toss until heated thoroughly. Salt and pepper to taste.

Makes 6 1 cup servings

## Recipe Notes

*Braggs is an all natural alternative to soy sauce. It doesn't contain any alcohol or preservatives. The ingredients are: Vegetable protein from soybeans and purified water only. This makes it Daniel Fast Friendly :) You will be amazed at how closely it tastes like soy sauce!*

*Where to buy it: I have found it at Wal-Mart next to the soy sauce. I have also found it at many other stores in the organic, natural foods section.*

# Vegetable Lo Mein

*1 8oz.* box whole-grain spaghetti noodles
*1* large Chinese cabbage, shredded -cut into thin strips
*1* cup onion, chopped
*2* cups shredded carrot
*1* can bean sprouts, drained and rinsed
*1* can sliced water chestnuts, drained and rinsed
*1* can bamboo shoots, drained and rinsed
*1* cup pea pods, cut in 4 pieces
*1* bunch green onion, diced
*1* whole ginger root, 2 in. long cut into 8 pieces
*2* teaspoons minced garlic
*7* tablespoons Braggs (Alternative to Soy Sauce)
*1/2* cup water
*1/2* teaspoon red pepper flakes
*4* tablespoons peanut oil
*2* tablespoons sesame oil
Hoisin Sauce (recipe follows)

### Instructions
- Cook the spaghetti noodles as directed on the package. Drain and toss with 2 Tablespoons of Sesame oil, set aside.
- Shred the cabbage (cut into strips), and carrot (can use pre-shredded carrots). Place in a large bowl.
- Drain and rinse bean sprouts, water chestnuts, bamboo shoots and add to the shredded vegetables
- Cut up the pea pods, and add to bowl of vegetables. Set aside
- Chop onion using the Vidalia chopper coarse insert, cut up green onion. Place both onions aside.

- Prepare Hoisin Sauce, set aside.
- Place the fresh ginger and garlic in the food processor and blend. Put the ginger and garlic mixture in a small bowl and set aside.
- In a separate small bowl, mix 3 heaping tablespoons of Hoisin sauce, water, pepper flakes, Braggs, sesame oil. Set aside

Now you are ready to make some INCREDIBLE Lo mein!

- Heat Peanut oil over medium heat. Add ginger garlic mixture, green and regular onions, stir for 1 minute
- Add all the vegetables and stir fry for 4 minutes
- Stirring constantly, add noodles and the Hoisin Sauce mixture and toss well
- Heat for about 2 to 3 minutes tossing until heated through

### Hoisin Sauce

*6* tablespoons Braggs (Alternative to Soy Sauce)
*2* tablespoons lemon juice
*2* tablespoons peanut butter, natural
*2* tablespoons Agave nectar
*2* tablespoons sesame oil
*1/2* teaspoon red pepper flakes
*2* teaspoons garlic powder
*3* teaspoons five-spice powder
*10* whole pitted dried prunes, Sunsweet gold label

#### Instructions

- Put all the ingredients in a food processor and blend on high for 2-3 minutes until prunes are small specks

# Oriental Eggplant

*1* pound oriental eggplant (cut in half and then in ½ inch circles)
*3* tablespoons peanut oil
*1* teaspoon chopped garlic
*1/4* teaspoon red pepper flakes
*6* whole green onions, cut in circles
*1* tablespoon sesame oil
*1* tablespoon whole grain, whole wheat flour
*2* tablespoons Braggs (Alternative to Soy Sauce)
*3/4* cup vegetable broth
*2* tablespoons toasted sesame seeds

### Instructions

- For the Sauce mixture: In a small bowl, add sesame oil and flour ...stir to incorporate, then add Braggs and vegetable broth , stir and set aside.
- In a large skillet, on medium high heat, add peanut oil and eggplant. Sauté and stir for about 4 minutes
- Then add garlic, pepper flakes and green onions, continue stirring for about 2 more minutes
- Add sauce mixture. Stir until sauce becomes gravy like (about 1 minute)
- Place on serving dish and sprinkle with sesame seeds

Serves: 4.

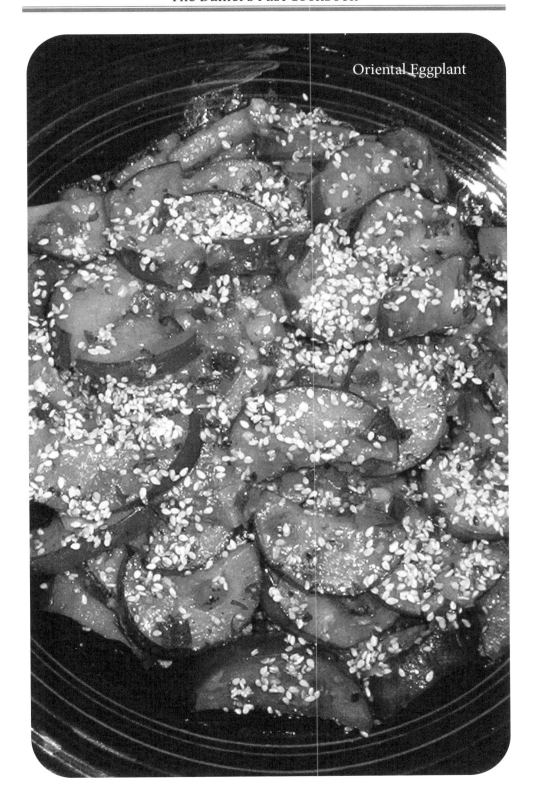

Oriental Eggplant

# Asian Pesto Spaghetti

*8* ounces Whole-grain spaghetti noodles, uncooked
*8* ounces shredded carrot, about 2 cups
*2* cups frozen peas
*1* cup cilantro leaves
*4* whole garlic cloves, peeled
*1 ½* whole ginger root, about 1.5 inches long, peeled
*3/4* cup green onion, chopped
*1/2* cup dry roasted cashew nut, use divided
*1/4* cup extra virgin olive oil
*2* teaspoons lemon juice
*1* teaspoon salt
*1/2* teaspoon pepper

### Instructions

- Cook spaghetti according to directions, adding carrots and peas during the last 2 minutes of cooking. RESERVE 1/2 CUP OF COOKING WATER for later use. Then DRAIN.
- Pour drained cooked pasta into a bowl. Set aside.
- Meanwhile, in food processor, puree' garlic, cilantro, ginger, green onions, olive oil, cashews, lemon juice, salt and pepper until smooth.
- Then add cooking water (if you forget the pasta water ..just add hot water).
- Toss spaghetti with cilantro mixture
- Chop remaining cashews and sprinkle over the top
- Salt and pepper to taste.

May be served hot or at room temp.

### Recipe Notes

*Family Friendly suggestion: Sauté 1 lb raw peeled*

*de veined shrimp in olive oil and add to family's portion. I like the frozen raw ready to cook 26 to 30 size.*
***Short cuts****: Use the pre-shredded carrots in the produce aisle. Fresh Lemon Juice can be found in the freezer section.*

Serves: 4.

# Japanese Cabbage Salad

*1* 16 oz. package Shredded Cabbage Trio (white, purple cabbage w/carrots)
*1* 8 oz. package of whole grain pasta (no egg), cooked & drained
*1* 8 oz. can bamboo shoots, drained and rinsed
*1* 8 oz. can sliced water chestnuts, drained and rinsed
*1/4* pound pea pods, cut in 4 pieces
Ginger Garlic Japanese Dressing (recipe on following page)

### Instructions
- Mix all the ingredients together in a large bowl.
- Pour the Ginger Garlic Japanese Dressing over the salad and toss.
- Salt and pepper to taste.

### Recipe Notes
*You can use frozen peas in place of the pea pods.*
*This salad keeps well in the refrigerator for up to four days.*

# Ginger Garlic Japanese Dressing

*3* tablespoons lemon juice
*3* tablespoons peanut oil
*3* tablespoons sesame oil
*3* teaspoons chopped garlic
*1* whole ginger root, 3 in. long peeled and chopped
*5* teaspoons Braggs (Alternative to Soy Sauce)
*1 ½* teaspoons pepper

## *Instructions*

- Place all ingredients into food processor and blend for 2 minutes.

Keep in refrigerator for 1 week.

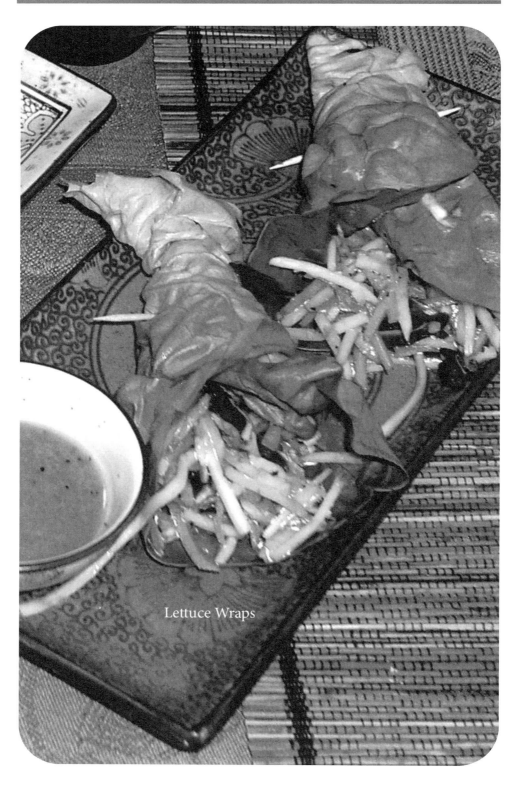

Lettuce Wraps

# Lettuce Wraps

*4* bibb Lettuce Leaves
*1* cup Broccoli slaw
Ginger Garlic Japanese Dressing (recipe follows)

### Instructions

- Mix the broccoli slaw with 1/4 cup ginger garlic Japanese dressing
- Salt and pepper to taste.
- Fill each bibb leaf with 1/4 cup slaw mixture and secure with a toothpick. Enjoy!

### Recipe Notes

*IF you have left over Japanese Cabbage Salad, you can use it to fill the bibb leaves instead of the broccoli slaw.*
*The Broccoli Slaw is made by Mann's and can be found in the bagged salad section at most general grocery stores.*

# Ginger Garlic Japanese Dressing

*3* tablespoons lemon juice
*3* tablespoons peanut oil
*3* tablespoons sesame oil
*3* teaspoons chopped garlic
*1* whole ginger root, 3 in. long peeled and chopped
*5* teaspoons Braggs (Alternative to Soy Sauce)
*1 ½* teaspoons pepper

### Instructions

- Place all ingredients into food processor and blend for 2minutes.

Keep in refrigerator for 1 week.

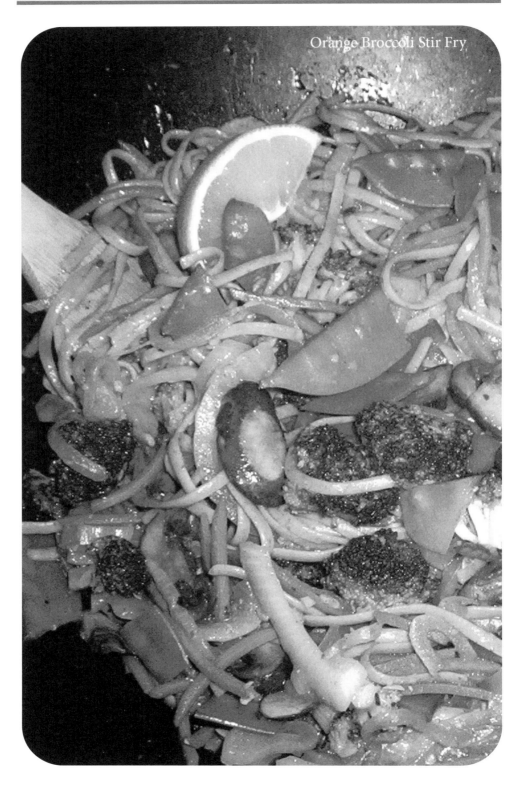

Orange Broccoli Stir Fry

# Orange Broccoli Stir Fry

*1* 8 oz pkg. of whole wheat linguine, drained & tossed w/ olive oil

*2* tablespoons olive oil

*1* 10 oz. pkg. of sliced baby bella mushrooms

*1 ½* cups shredded carrot

*1* large sweet onion cut in half, then thin slices

*1* tablespoon chopped garlic

*3* cups broccoli florets

*20* whole snow pea pods, cut in 3 pieces at an angle

Orange Broccoli Stir Fry Sauce (recipe follows)

### Instructions

- In a large wok or pan, add the olive oil. On high heat, sauté the onions for about two minutes stirring constantly
- Add mushrooms and sauté for two more minutes
- Then add the remaining ingredients
- Stir for several minutes
- Then turn down to medium heat and cover for 3 minutes
- Then add the sauce and stir until mixed well
- On high heat continue to stir until thickened
- Add linguine to mixture and toss, remove from heat...it's time to eat!

# Orange Broccoli Stir Fry Sauce

*2* tablespoons sesame oil
*2* tablespoons whole grain, whole wheat flour
*1* teaspoon Chinese five spice powder
*1/2* teaspoon red pepper flakes
*1* cup orange juice
*4* tablespoons Braggs (Alternative to Soy Sauce)
*1* zest of one orange

### Instructions
- Put the sesame seed oil in a small bowl, add flour and whisk together
- Then add remaining ingredients and whisk again.

This recipe was created for the Orange Broccoli Stir Fry recipe. However you can use this sauce on any of your favorite stir fry's

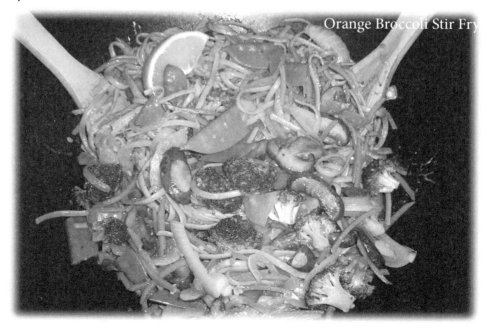

Orange Broccoli Stir Fry

# Chili Garlic Paste

*1* tablespoon of tomato paste
*1* teaspoon of powder garlic,
*1/2* teaspoon of red pepper flakes
*3* tablespoon of sesame seed oil
*3* tablespoon of Braggs (alternative to soy sauce)

**Recipe Instructions**
Mix all these ingredients in a small bowl and set aside

**Recipe Notes**
*This recipe was created for the Oriental Baby Pasta Recipe.*

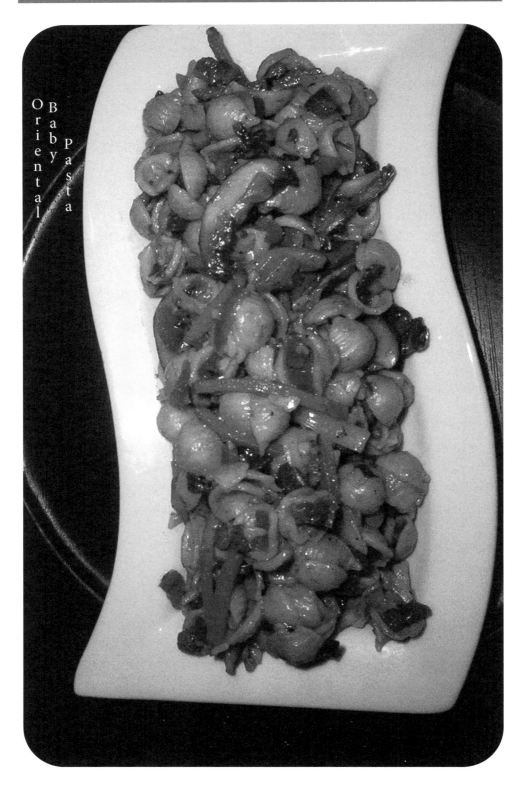

Oriental Baby Pasta

# Oriental Baby Pasta

*1* 16 oz. package of whole wheat baby sea shell pasta, cooked & drained
*1* tablespoon olive oil
*1* cup shredded carrot
*1* 10 oz. pkg. of sliced baby bella mushrooms
*1/2* cup green bell pepper, chopped w/Vidalia fine insert
*1* whole red onion, chopped w/Vidalia fine insert
*1* teaspoon ground ginger
*1* bunch green onion, sliced thin
*1/2* bunch cilantro leaves, chopped fine
*1* teaspoon chopped garlic
*1* teaspoon salt
*1* teaspoon pepper
Chili Garlic Paste (recipe on previous page)

### *Instructions*

- Make Chili Garlic paste and set aside.
- In a large pan on high heat, place olive oil, onions, bell peppers, mushrooms, carrots and sauté for about 4 minutes stirring constantly, add ginger, garlic , green onions, salt and pepper and chili paste
- Stir for about 2 minutes, add cilantro and cooked baby pasta
- Combine all together well and serve room temperature or cold.

Serves: 4.

# Mongolian Vegetables

*2* tablespoons peanut oil

*1* large head of bok choy (white only), sliced in ½ inch circles

*1* large red bell pepper, cut in thin strips

*1* bunch green onion, cut in circles

*2* cups snow pea pods

*1* 8 oz. can sliced water chestnuts, drained and rinsed

*1* 14.5 oz. can of bean sprouts, drained and rinsed

*2* teaspoons chopped garlic

*2* tablespoons sesame oil

*2* tablespoons whole grain, whole wheat flour

*5* tablespoons Braggs (Alternative to Soy Sauce)

*1/2* teaspoon pepper

*1 ½* cups vegetable broth

## *Instructions*

- In a small bowl, mix the sesame oil and flour together
- Then add Braggs, pepper and stock...mix well and set aside.
- In a large skillet place, 2 tbsp of peanut oil, add red bell pepper and bok choy, sauté for about 3 min
- Then add pea pods, green onions and chopped garlic. Continue sautéing for another 3 minutes
- Then add bean sprouts and water chestnuts, toss around and cook for another minute
- Then add sauce mixture, stirring constantly until it thickens
- Let bubble for a few more minutes ...if desired, serve over whole grain brown rice

Serves: 4.

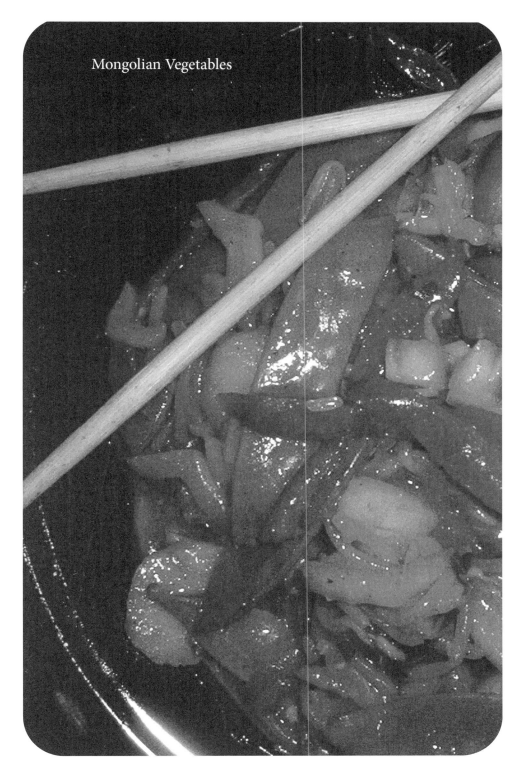

Mongolian Vegetables

# Mexican Dishes

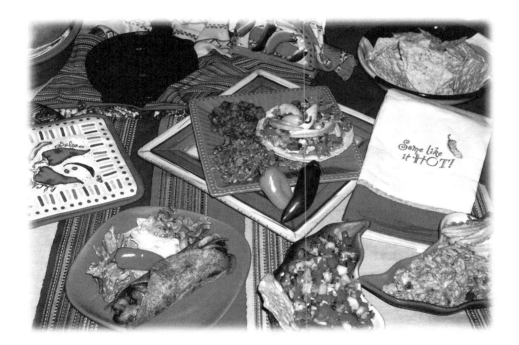

# Mexican Rice

*1* cup whole grain brown rice, uncooked
*2 ½* cups cold water
*2* tablespoons olive oil
*1* cup white onion, diced
*2* tablespoons garlic cloves, minced
*1* 14.5 oz. can diced tomatoes
*1/2* whole green bell pepper, diced
*1 ½* teaspoons salt
*1* teaspoon pepper
*1 ½* teaspoon cumin

### Instructions

- Using a frying pan with a lid, add olive oil and rice.
- Over medium high heat, stir the rice to a golden brown.
- Then add garlic,2 1/2 cups cold water and the can of tomatoes.
- Bring to a boil and reduce to low heat.
- Add remaining ingredients stir and cover. Let cook for 1 hour 15 min...check after 45 minutes as temperature and time varies with each stove...Prior to that....don't peek!
- Uncover and remove from heat, let sit for 5 minutes

### Recipe Notes

When it is ready, all the water will be absorbed, the rice will fluff, it shouldn't be dry or not too saucy.

Serves: 4.

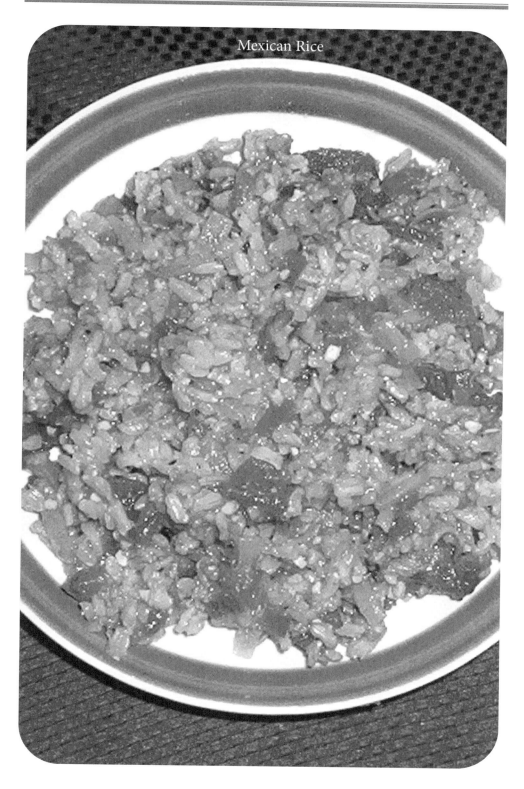

Mexican Rice

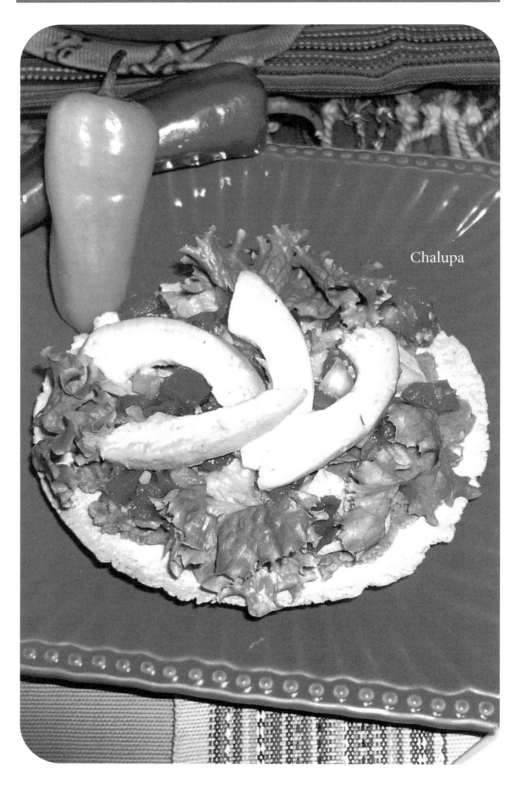

Chalupa

# Chalupas

Corn Tortilla (recipe follows)
Simple Salsa (recipe follows)
Guacamole (recipe follows)
Refried beans (recipe follows)
1/2 head Lettuce, shredded -cut into thin strips

## Instructions
- Preheat the oven to 375°
- Place corn tortillas on a cookie sheet and bake for 5-10 minutes or until hard.
- Smear on warm refried beans.
- Pile on the lettuce then scoop on the Salsa and Guacamole. Enjoy!

## Recipe Notes
Short cuts:
Whole Foods Market makes an organic corn tortilla that doesn't contain anything but corn and water. They can be found in the refrigerator section. Most other brands contain ingredients NO-NOs.

You can also buy vegetarian refried beans. And instead of making Guacamole, you can simply cut an avocado on top. Some stores sell fresh Pica de Gallo (salsa) in containers near the bagged salads. They usually contain safe ingredients.

Also, you can pick up pre-shredded lettuce in the bagged salad area at the store.

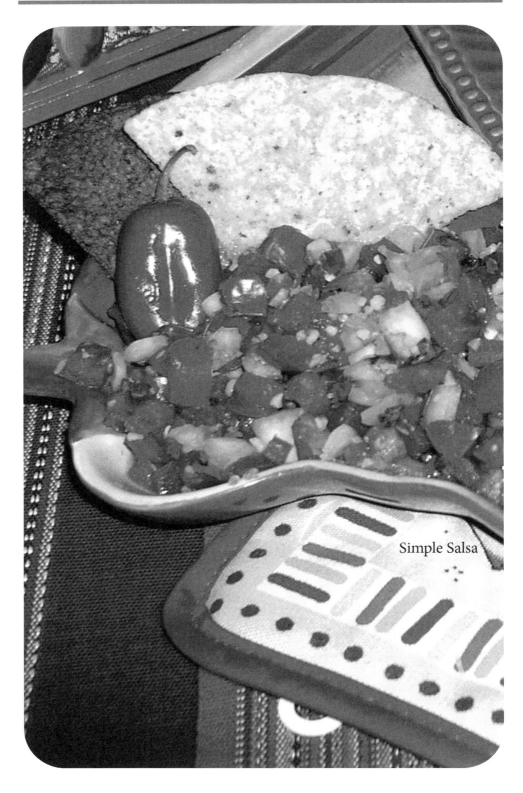

Simple Salsa

# Simple Salsa

*5* whole roma tomatoes, diced
*1/2* whole white onion, diced
*1* whole jalapeno pepper, diced fine
*1/2* cup cilantro leaves, torn
*1* tablespoon chopped garlic, jar ok
*1* tablespoon of lemon juice
*1/2* teaspoon black pepper
*1* teaspoon salt

### Instructions

- Use the Vidalia Chop Wizard coarse insert to dice the Roma tomatoes and onion, place in a large bowl.
- Use the small dice insert of the chop wizard to finely dice the jalapeno, add to the tomatoes and onion.
- Next add, the cilantro leaves, lemon juice, chopped garlic, pepper and salt.
- Stir until mixed well. Makes 3 cups

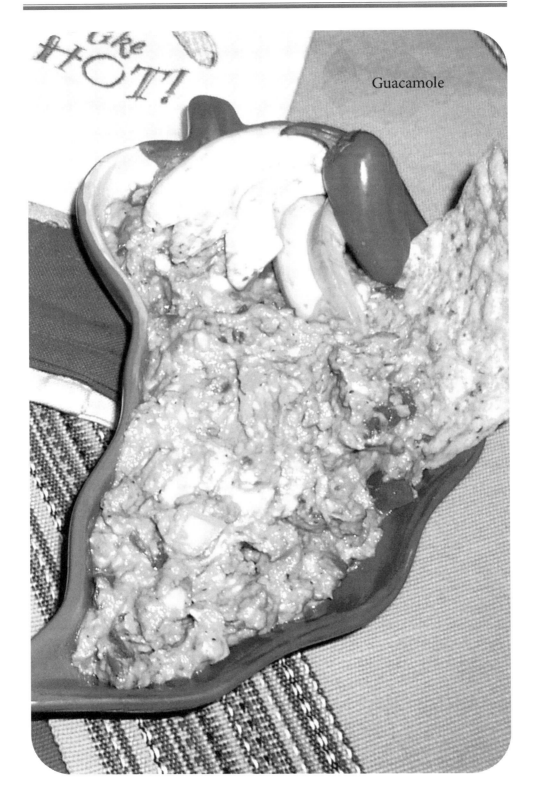

Guacamole

# Guacamole

*4* large avocados, (about 6 average sized)
*1* whole juice of a lime
*1/2* teaspoon salt
*1/2* teaspoon pepper
*1/2* cup of Simple Salsa (recipe on previous page)

### Instructions

- Slice avocados in half, removing the skin and pits. Cut off dark spots and place in a bowl
- Add 1/2 cup of the Simple Salsa, lime juice, salt and pepper. Mash well. Makes 4 cups.

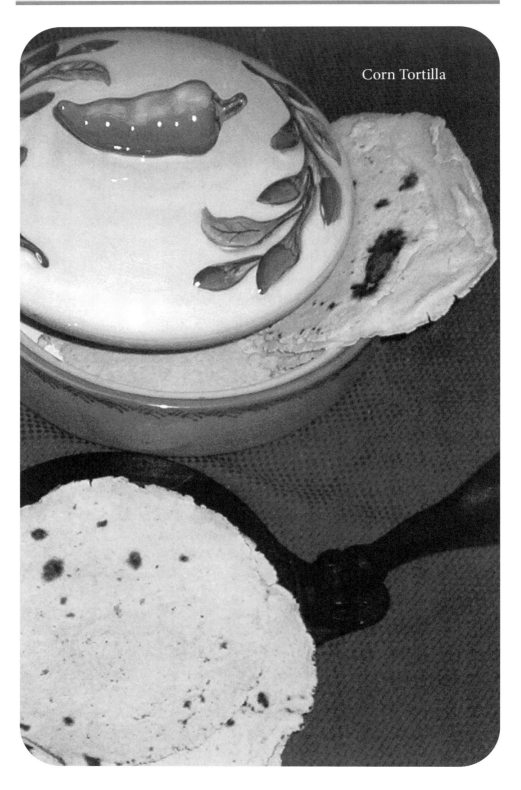

Corn Tortilla

# Corn Tortilla

*2* cups Masa corn flour
*1 ¼* cups water
*1/2* teaspoon salt

## Instructions

- Mix the masa, salt and water together in a large bowl. The mixture should stick together...but it should not be too sticky or crumbly. If it is crumbly add 1 tablespoon of water at a time until the desired consistency is accomplished.
- Form into 3 in. balls (a little larger than a golf ball).
- Now its time to press them. You will need a tortilla press and a quart size Ziploc bag. (I like to use the zip loc bags instead of wax paper)
- Cut the zip loc bag along the seems...so you will have too square pieces.
- Place the ball in between the Ziploc bag pieces on the tortilla press and firmly press down.
-  Peel the tortilla away from the Ziploc bag
- Cook on a hot griddle, about 2 minutes on each side.

This makes 8-10 tortillas

## Recipe Notes

*A tortilla press can be purchased online for about $20, I have also seen them at World Market.*
*Do not use corn meal... it is not the same and it will not work.*

Serves: 8.

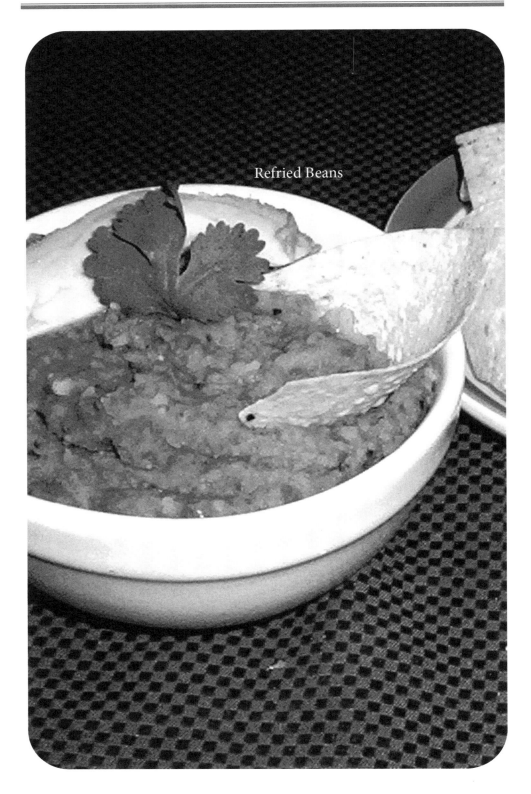

Refried Beans

# Refried beans

Mexican Pinto Beans (recipe follows)
*1/8* teaspoon garlic powder
*1/2* teaspoon salt
*1/2* teaspoon cumin
*1/2* cup white onion, chopped
*3* tablespoons olive oil
*1/3* cup water

### Instructions

- In a food processor, add 2 cups of Mexican Pinto Beans, 1/3 cup of water, 1/8 teaspoon of garlic powder, salt and cumin.  Blend on med-high until creamy.
- In a frying pan, over medium-high heat, fry onion in olive oil.  When onions are clear, add the creamed pinto beans.
- Sauté for about 5 minutes, until desired consistency is reached.  Keep in mind, the beans will thicken as they cool.

Makes 2 cups of refried beans..

### Recipe Notes
*Refried beans are great for bean burritos, Chalupas and dip for whole-grain corn chips.*
*I made a big batch and freeze extra portions.*

A full recipe of Mexican Pinto Beans makes about 8 cups of pinto beans. So if desired, repeat the above directions until all beans have been used

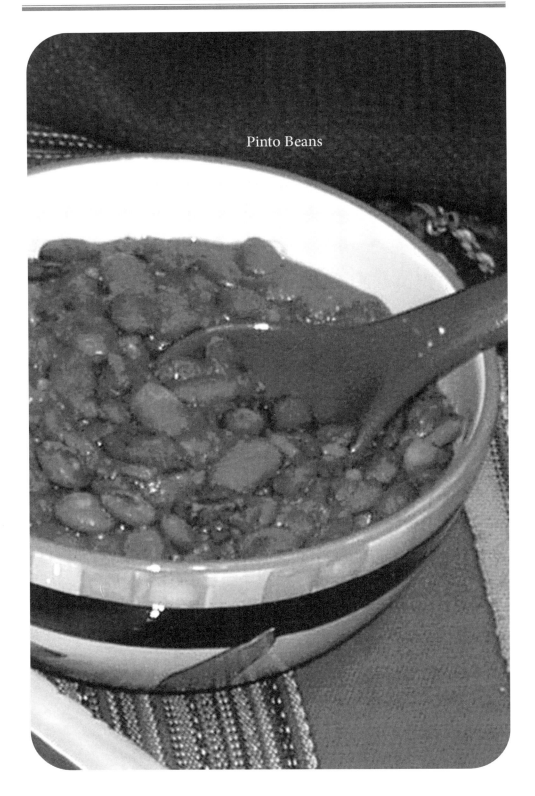

Pinto Beans

# Mexican Pinto Beans

*1* pound pinto bean, dried (approx 2 cups)
*6* cups water
*1* teaspoon cumin
*1/2* teaspoon salt
*1/4* teaspoon garlic powder
*1/4* teaspoon onion powder
*1/8* teaspoon chili powder

## Instructions

- Look through the beans for rocks and foreign matter, rinse.
- Add enough water to cover the beans about 2 inches.
- Soak overnight or bring to a boil for 3 min and then turn off heat and let sit for 4 hours.
- Drain the soaking water from the beans and place them in a slow cooker (crock pot).
- Add enough fresh water to cover the beans with about 1 inch (approx 6 cups)
- Cook at a low setting for 6-8 hours.
- 30 min before serving add seasonings and simmer

If you do not have a crock pot

- Place the pre-soaked beans in a pot and cover with 1 inch of fresh water (approx 6)
- Bring to a boil then reduce the heat and simmer on low for 2 1/2 hours or until beans are tender.
- Add the seasoning 30 min before serving and simmer.

## Recipe Notes

*Do not let the beans dry out. Add water as needed and stir occasionally.*

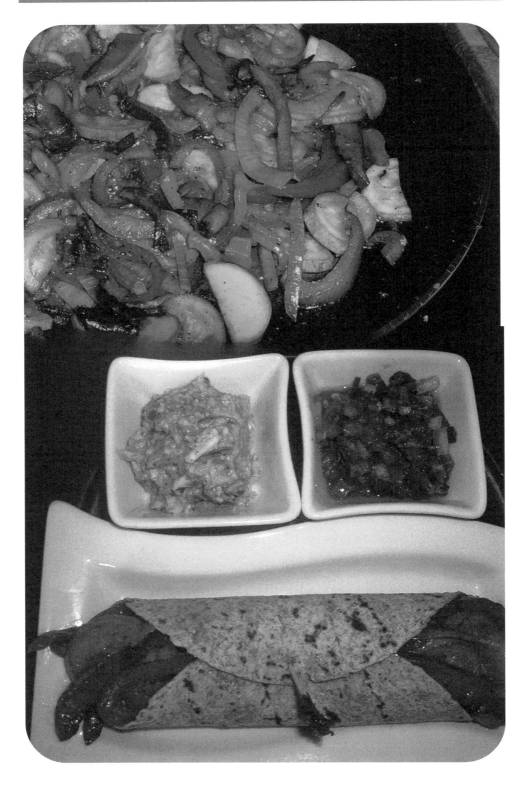

# Nada Asada

1 whole green bell pepper, sliced in 1/8" sl
3 whole portabella mushrooms, stem & gill
1 whole purple onion, cut in half, then thin
1 teaspoon chopped garlic
1/2 teaspoon salt
1/2 teaspoon pepper
1 teaspoon cumin
1 teaspoon chili powder
3 tablespoons olive oil
4 whole wheat, whole grain tortillas
2 whole zucchini, sliced in half moons about 1/8 inch thick

## Instructions

- In a non-stick skillet, get the olive oil hot and add onions, bell peppers and zucchini
- Continue to sauté on high heat stirring constantly
- After about 3 minutes add mushrooms and continue to cook for another 2 minutes
- Add garlic and all other seasonings and stir on med-high heat until vegetables are tender (just a few minutes)
- Remove from heat
- In a small pan, heat tortillas for about 20 to 30 seconds on each side
- Fill with Asada mixture and serve with salsa and guacamole

## Recipe Notes:

Serves: 4.

# Italian Dishes

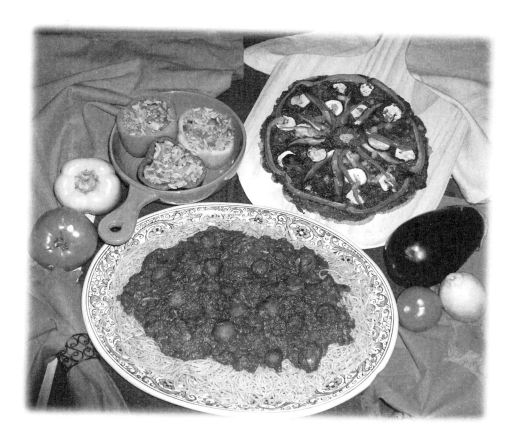

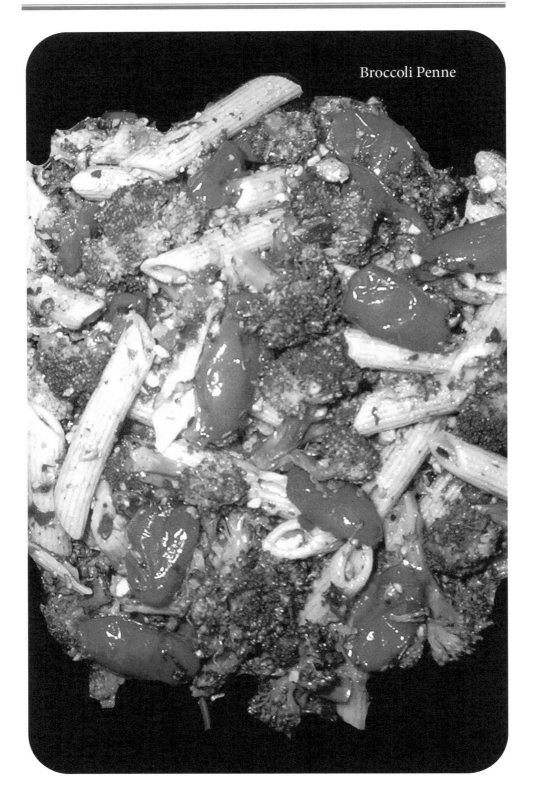

Broccoli Penne

# Broccoli Penne

*1* 8 oz. box whole wheat penne pasta, cooked per box instructions
*1/4* cup pasta water, reserved from cooking pasta
*1* 12 oz. package of Mann's Broccoli Wokley (in a microwave bag)
*4* whole sun-dried tomatoes in olive oil
*1* bunch flat leaf parsley
*4* tablespoons olive oil
*1* tablespoon chopped garlic, jar ok
*18* whole grape tomatoes, cut in half
*1/4* teaspoon red pepper flakes
*1* teaspoon salt
*1* teaspoon pepper
*1/4* cup pistachio nuts, crushed

### Instructions

- Using a fork, poke a hole in top of the broccoli wokley bag and place in the microwave for 4 min on high.
- Remove and open bag carefully and set aside.
- In the food processor, put 4 sun dried tomatoes, 1 Tbsp of olive oil (from sun dried tomato jar), flat leaf parsley and 4 Tbsp of reserved pasta water. Blend well for about 1 minute and set aside.
- In a large skillet, sauté olive oil and garlic for a minute, then add tomatoes for just 2 more minutes over medium heat.
- Add sun dried tomato mixture, cooked broccoli and cooked penne
- Toss to blend. Heat for just a few minutes ..sprinkle pistachio nuts over the top and serve.

**Recipe Notes:**

*The Mann's Broccoli Wokley can be found in the produce section by the salads. If you can't find Mann's broccoli, simply use any cooked broccoli of your choosing.*

Serves: 4.

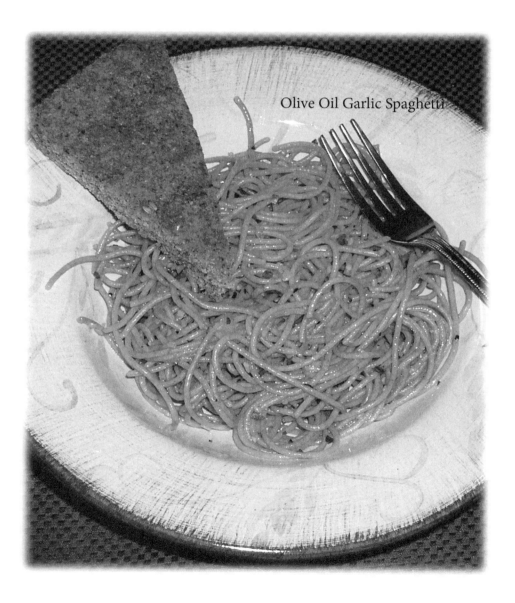

Olive Oil Garlic Spaghetti

# Olive Oil Garlic Spaghetti

*1* pound whole-grain spaghetti noodles, cooked and drained
*1/2* cup olive oil
*3* tablespoons minced garlic, jar ok
*1/4* teaspoon red pepper flakes
*3* teaspoons minced onions (fresh)
Salt & pepper to taste

### *Instructions*
- Heat oil in large frying skillet and add garlic and onion
- Sauté over medium heat for about 5 minutes or until golden brown.  Be careful not to burn.
- Add red pepper, fresh ground pepper and salt to taste
- Put the cooked spaghetti in with the oil/garlic mixture and toss ...let pasta warm up for a few minutes

Simple but sooooo good!

Serves: 6.

*Pictured with the Italian Flat Bread

# Baby Portabella Mushroom Marinara Sauce

*2* 8 oz. packages of whole Baby Portabella mushrooms
*1* 12. oz bag of frozen chopped onions
*2* tablespoons minced garlic, jar ok
*2* 28 oz. cans crushed tomatoes with Italian Herbs
*1* 6 oz. can tomato paste
*1* tablespoon olive oil
*1* packet stevia
*2* teaspoons dried basil
*1* teaspoon dried oregano
*1* teaspoon fennel seed
*1* teaspoon pepper
*1*teaspoon salt
*1* teaspoon red pepper flakes

## *Instructions*

- Mix all ingredients in a 3 1/2 to 4 quart slow cooker(crock pot).
- Cover and cook on low heat setting for 6 to 8 hours. Stirring occasionally.

Serve sauce over whole wheat spaghetti (no eggs).

If you do not have a slow cooker (crock pot)
- Put all the ingredients in a medium sauce pan and bring to a boil.
- Reduce heat and simmer for 45 min.

The sauce tastes better if it can simmer in a slow cooker for 6-8 hours.

## *Recipe Notes*

*Family Friendly Version: Have family not on the Fast? Brown up 1 lb of ground chuck and 1 lb of Italian sausage, drain and add to the Marinara Sauce after taking out for yourself.*

*If you can't find the Italian herb crushed tomatoes, use the plain and add an additional 1/2 teaspoon of oregano, 1/2 teaspoon of basil and 1/2 teaspoon of garlic powder.*

*Also, if you don't like spicy food leave out the red pepper flakes they add a little heat.*

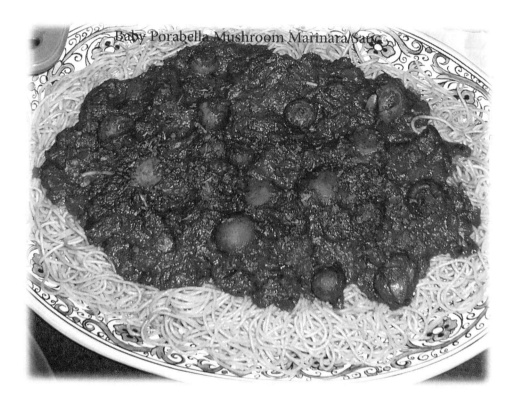

Baby Porabella Mushroom Marinara Sauce

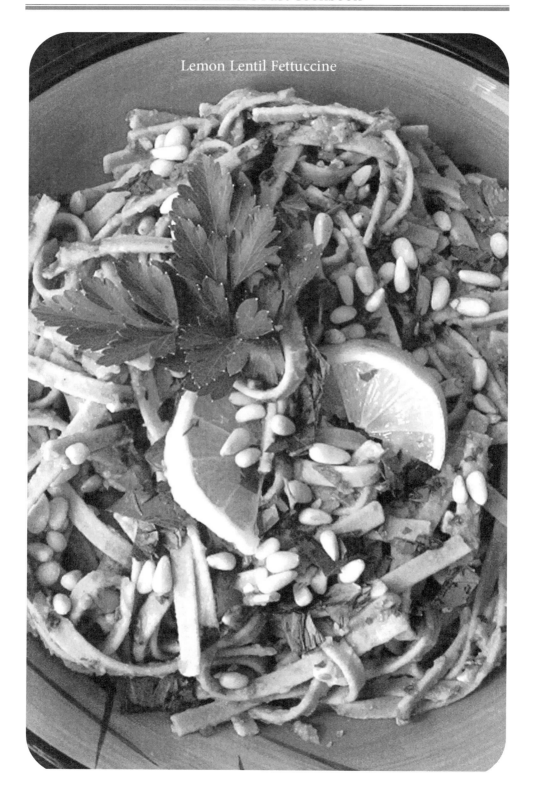

Lemon Lentil Fettuccine

# Lemon Lentil Fettuccine

*1* 12 oz. box whole wheat fettuccine
*2* 15 oz. can lentils, reserving 1/4 cup of juice
*1/4* cup olive oil
*1/4* cup lemon juice
*2* teaspoons chopped garlic, jar ok
*1/2* cup flat leaf parsley, chopped
*3/4* cup toasted pine nuts, reserve 1/4 cup for garnish
*2* teaspoons salt
*1* teaspoon pepper

### Instructions
- Cook the fettuccine according to the boxes instructions.
- While the fettuccine is cooking, place all ingredients in the food processor including 1/4 cup of lentil juice. Blend until smooth, but still has texture.
- Pour into large pasta bowl and set aside.
-  After draining fettuccine noodles, dump in the pasta bowl and toss with lentil mixture.
- Garnish with chopped parsley and toasted pine nuts.
- Serve immediately.

### Recipe Notes
*To toast the pine nuts, Pre heat the oven to 350°.  Spread the nuts on an ungreased shallow pan and bake for 10 min. Stir occasionally.*

Serves: 6.

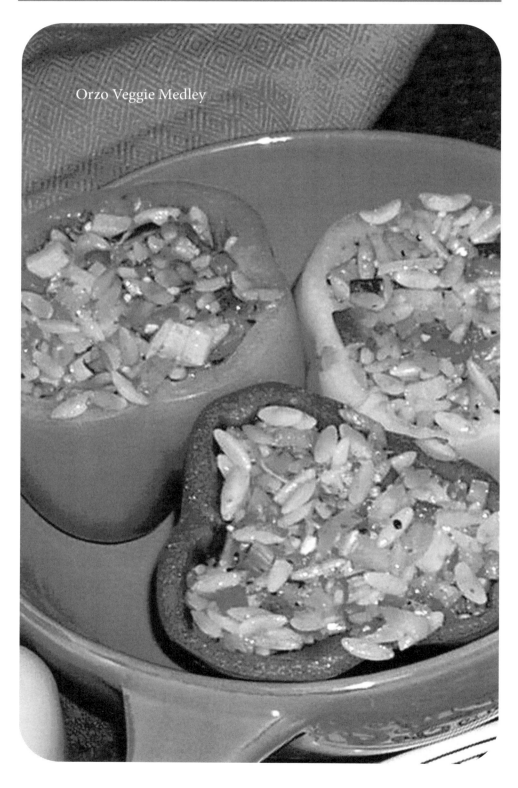

Orzo Veggie Medley

# Orzo Veggie Medley

*1* cup Orzo, (whole wheat & no eggs)
*2* tablespoons olive oil
*1* teaspoon garlic, finely chopped
*1* teaspoon lemon juice, freshly squeezed
*1/2* teaspoon pepper
*1/2* teaspoon salt
*1* pinch dried thyme leaves
*1* whole zucchini, w/Vidalia chopper fine insert
*3* ribs celery, w/Vidalia chopper fine insert
*1/2* cup leek, w/Vidalia chopper fine insert
*2* tablespoons fennel bulbs, w/Vidalia chopper fine insert
*2* whole tomatoes, chopped, w/Vidalia chopper fine insert
*1/4* cup yellow bell pepper, w/Vidalia chopper fine insert
1/4 cup red bell pepper, w/Vidalia chopper fine insert

### Instructions

- Bring 2 quarts of water to a boil. Slowly add orzo, boil for 5 min.
- Drain and set aside. Orzo should be al dente.
- Chop all the vegetables with the small Vidalia chopper insert. In a sauté pan, combine all other ingredients and sauté over medium high heat for 8 min.
- Toss in Orzo and continue to sauté for a couple of minutes.

Can be served in Bell Pepper or Tomato boats.

### Recipe Notes

*When choosing an Orzo, make sure it does not contain any animal products including egg. Most Orzo is simple pasta containing flour and water.*

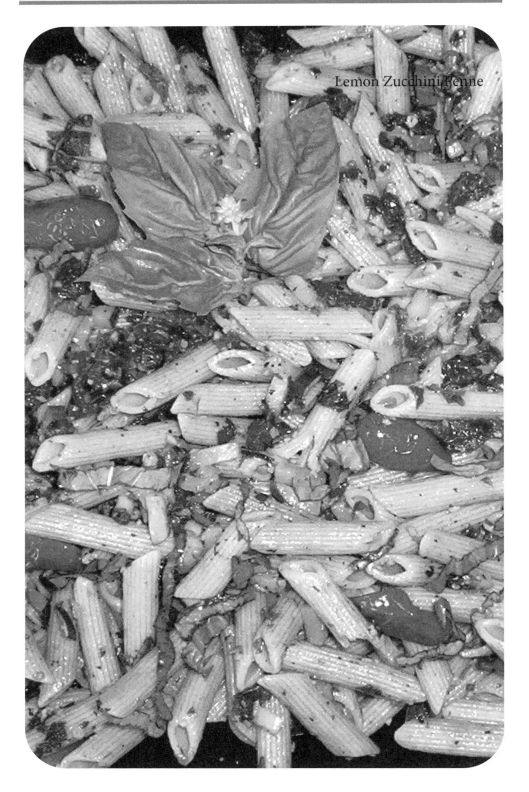

Lemon Zucchini Penne

# Lemon Zucchini Penne

*1* 12 oz. box of whole wheat penne, cooked per box instructions
*1/4* cup olive oil
*1/2* teaspoon red pepper flakes, crushed
*2* teaspoons chopped garlic, jar ok
*1* large zucchini chopped w/Vidalia fine insert, about 1 cup
*12* whole grape tomatoes, cut in half
*10* whole sun-dried tomatoes in olive oil, cut into bits
*1/2* cup chopped flat leaf parsley
1teaspoon dried basil
*1/4* cup lemon juice
*1* teaspoon salt
*1* teaspoon pepper

### Recipe Notes

- In a pan, sauté olive oil, red pepper flakes, garlic and zucchini for about 5 minutes on medium heat stirring constantly.
- Then add grape tomatoes and dried tomatoes, parsley, basil, salt, pepper and lemon juice.
- Cook for an additional five minutes. Then add cooked, drained penne to pan and combine well. Serve warm.

Serves: 4

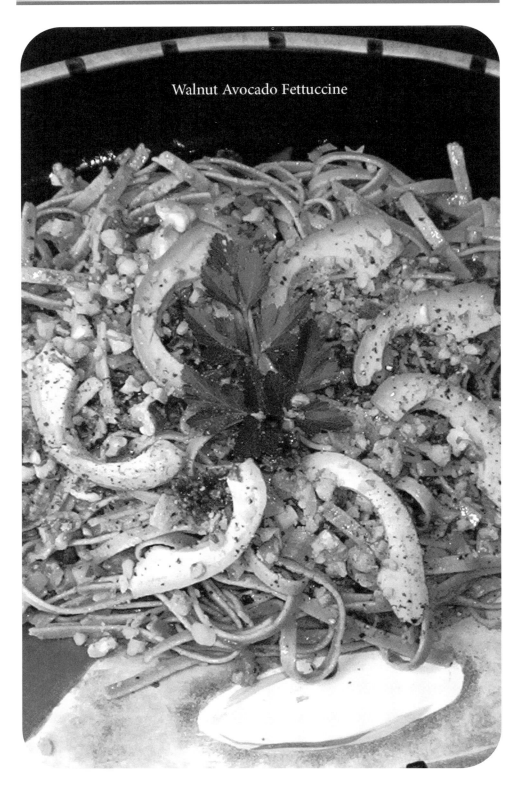

Walnut Avocado Fettuccine

# Walnut Avocado Fettuccine

*1* 12 oz. box of whole wheat penne, cooked per box instructions
*4* tablespoons olive oil
*2* teaspoons chopped garlic, jar ok
*1/4* cup lemon juice
*10* whole sun-dried tomatoes in olive oil
*1* cup green pepper, chopped w/Vidalia fine insert
*1* cup walnuts, chopped
*2* whole avocadoes diced, save 1/2 avocado for garnish
*1/2* cup green onion, chopped
*1* teaspoon salt
*1* teaspoon pepper

### Instructions

- Start the water boiling for the fettuccine.
- In the meantime, in a large bowl place olive oil, garlic and lemon juice and whisk together.
- Then add remaining ingredients reserving 1/4 cup walnuts and 1/2 avocado for garnish.
- Stir with a spoon until everything is combined well...set aside and continue with cooking the fettuccine.
- After draining the noodles, add them to the olive oil mixture and toss well
- Serve on a platter, garnish with avocado slices and walnuts... This dish may be served warm or at room temperature

Serves: 6.

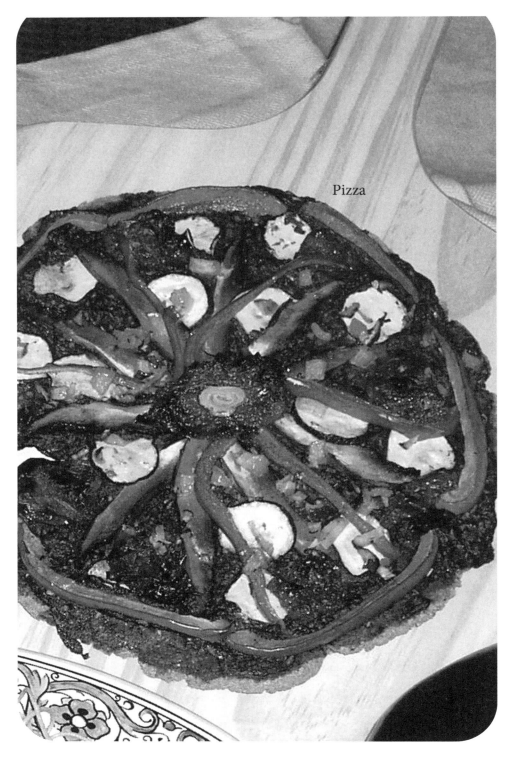

Pizza

# Pizza

Pizza Sauce (recipe on follows)
Whole Grain Pizza Crust (recipe follows)
1 whole zucchini, sliced
1/2 whole red bell pepper, chopped
5 whole sun-dried tomatoes in olive oil
1/4 whole red onion, sliced
1 6 oz sliced fresh sliced mushrooms

### Instructions
- Preheat oven to 375°
- Prepare pizza sauce and crust (recipes follow)
- Arrange your favorite vegetables on top and bake for 30 min or until crust is crispy.

The vegetables suggested make a delicious pizza

## Pizza Sauce
1 6 oz. can tomato paste
3 tablespoons minced garlic, jar ok
3 tablespoons Italian seasoning
1 teaspoon fennel seed
2 tablespoons olive oil
1/4 cup water
1 pinch salt

### Instructions
- Mix all the ingredients together and let sit for 30 min.

This is a good time to make the Pizza crust.

### Recipe Notes
*You can make this sauce and keep it in the refrigerator for up to seven days.*

**Whole Grain Pizza Crust**

*2* cups whole grain, whole wheat flour

*1/3* cup olive oil

*1* cup water

*1* teaspoon Italian seasoning

*1/2* teaspoon salt

*1* teaspoon fennel seed

*1/4* teaspoon garlic powder

*1* tablespoon olive oil for pan

### *Instructions*

- Mix flour, salt and seasonings in a large bowl.
- Add oil and work into the flour well, until the oil and flour are combined.
- As you are mixing the dough with your hands, slowly add 1 cup of water. This should form a well behaved dough.
- Knead until smooth.. If too dry add small amounts of water(1 tablespoon at a time). If it is too sticky, add 1 tablespoon of flour at a time.
- Press into a greased cookie sheet to make one large pizza or roll out into individual sized pizzas. You can use a tortilla press to make small pizzas. Makes 6-8 individual sized pizzas

### *Recipe Notes*

For best results bake on a pizza stone at 375˚, until the crust is crispy. This takes about 30 minutes with toppings.

# Roasted Tomato and Vegetable Penne

*4* whole tomatoes, sliced
*2* tablespoons garlic cloves, chopped
*1* teaspoon salt
*1* teaspoon pepper
*1/2* whole onion, sliced in rings
*4* tablespoons olive oil
*1* 12oz. box Penne, whole wheat
*2* whole yellow squash, cut in chunks
*3* cups asparagus, frozen, cut in strips
*2* whole carrots, cut in thin sticks 2in long
*2* whole zucchini cut in thin sticks 2in long
*1/2* whole red bell pepper, cut in strips
*4* tablespoons olive oil
*2* tablespoons garlic cloves, diced
*1/2* teaspoon onion powder
*1* teaspoon pepper
*1/2* teaspoon red pepper flakes
*1* teaspoon salt

### Instructions
- Preheat the oven to 400°
- Place sliced tomatoes on a cookie sheet. Evenly spread diced garlic and olive oil on the top of the tomatoes.
- Sprinkle with salt, pepper. Cover the tomatoes with the sliced onion.
- Bake at 400° for 25-30 min.
- While the tomatoes are in the oven, cook the penne per the instructions on the box.
- Clean and cut all the vegetables.

- Over medium high heat, sauté all the vegetables with 4 Tbsp of olive oil.
- After 2 min add the garlic, onion powder, pepper and red pepper flakes.
- Continue to sauté for 5 more minutes. Add cooked penne and salt, stir until all the vegetables are mixed in.
- Add the roasted tomatoes and mix well. Serve warm

Serves: 6.

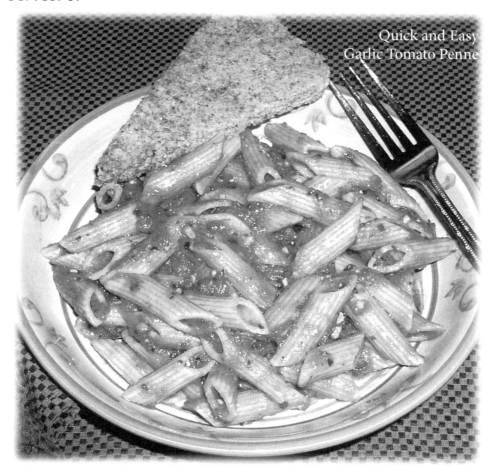

Quick and Easy Garlic Tomato Penne

# Quick and Easy Garlic, Tomato Penne

*1/2* cup olive oil
*2* tablespoons minced garlic, jar ok
*1* 28 oz. can crushed tomatoes with Italian herbs
*1* teaspoon red pepper flakes
*1/2* teaspoon salt
*1* tablespoon dried basil
*1* tablespoon dried parsley
*1* pound whole wheat (no egg) penne

### Instructions
- In a heavy sauce pan, heat olive oil and sauté garlic for about 2 minutes.
- Add red pepper flakes and tomatoes, salt, basil and parsley. Simmer uncovered on medium heat for about 20 minutes until liquid is almost gone
- With the back of your spoon mash the tomatoes. Toss in the cooked Penne, mix together well and continue to cook for 5 min..tossing several times.

### Recipe Notes
**Family Friendly Version**: *While sauce is cooking, fry 1 pound of Italian sausage and mix in with the penne for family's portion.*

Serves: 4.

# Simple Marinara Sauce

*1* 28 oz. can crushed tomatoes with Italian herbs
*2* 14.5 oz. can diced tomatoes with Italian seasonings
*2* cups white onions, diced
*1* 6 oz. can tomato paste
*2* tablespoons olive oil
*2* tablespoons minced garlic, jar ok
*1* packet stevia
*2* teaspoons dried basil
*1* teaspoon dried oregano
*1* teaspoon fennel seed
*1* teaspoon pepper
*1* teaspoon salt
*1* teaspoon red pepper flakes
*1* whole bay leaf

### Instructions

- Mix all ingredients in a 3 1/2 to 4 quart slow cooker(crock pot).
- Cover and cook on low heat setting for 4 hours. Stirring occasionally.

Before serving, take out the bay leaf. Serve sauce over whole wheat spaghetti (no eggs). Also goes great on spaghetti squash.(pictured on the following page)

If you do not have a slow cooker(crock pot)

- put all the ingredients in a medium sauce pan and bring to a boil.
- Reduce heat and simmer for 45 min.

### Recipe Notes

*Family Friendly Version*: Brown up 1 lb of ground chuck and 1 lb of Italian sausage. Drain and add to the Marinara Sauce after taking out for yourself.

*If you can't find the Italian herb crushed tomatoes, use the plain and add an additional 1/2 teaspoon of oregano, 1/2 teaspoon of basil and 1/2 teaspoon of garlic powder.*

Also, if you don't like spicy food leave out the red pepper flakes they add a little heat.

Spaghetti Squash is very simple to prepare.  Preheat the oven to 350° and cut the squash in half along the length. Remove the seeds and place in a dish cut side down.  Bake for 45 minutes.  Then simply scrape out the strands of squash.

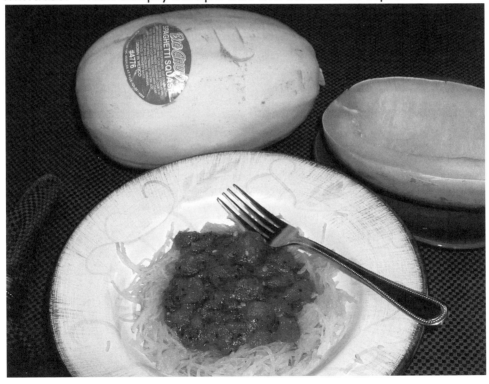

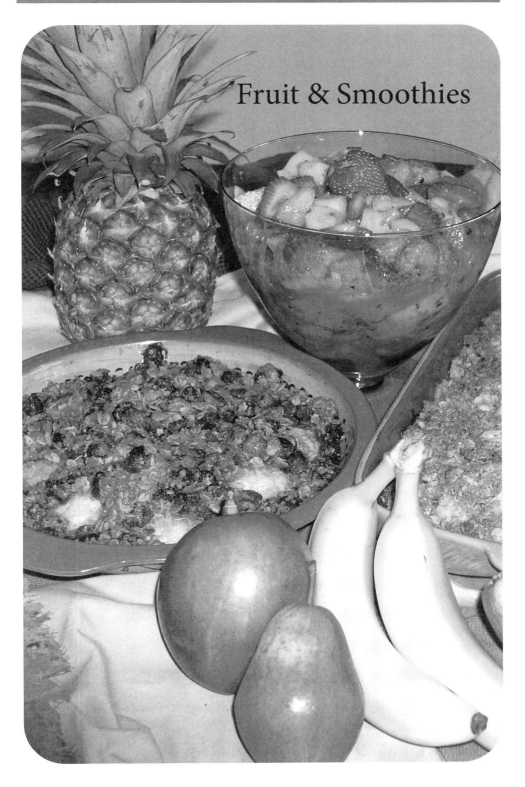

Fruit & Smoothies

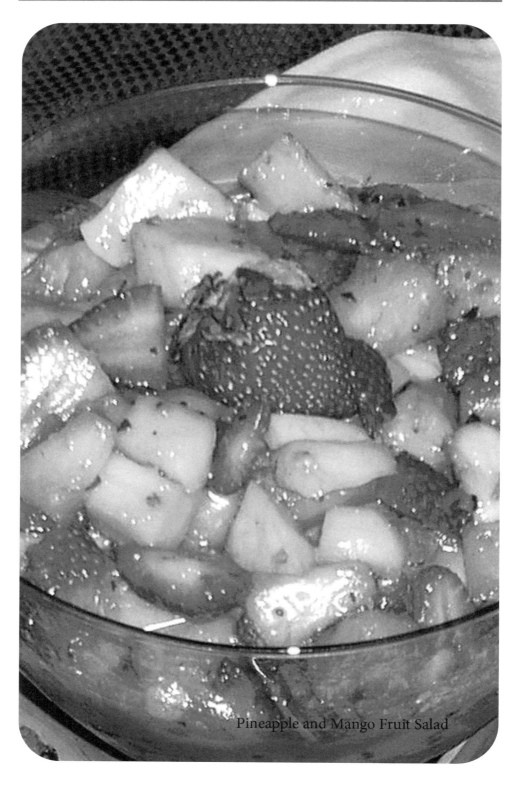

Pineapple and Mango Fruit Salad

# Pineapple and Mango Fruit Salad

*2* whole 16 oz. bags of frozen pineapple chunks (unsweetened)
*2* whole 12 oz bags of frozen mango chunks (unsweetened)
*1* whole 16 oz container of fresh strawberries
Cranberry-Orange Dressing (recipe on following page)

### Instructions
- Dump frozen fruit in a large bowl and let it semi-thaw ...about an hour.
- In the meantime, wash, remove stems and slice strawberries in two or larger three pieces and set aside.
- When the fruit is semi-thawed add the strawberries and Cranberry-Orange dressing.
-  Toss and serve cold

This will keep for three days in refrigerator.

### Recipe Notes
The frozen fruit can be purchased at Wal-mart. We recently purchased them for $1.56 a bag!

# Cranberry-Orange Dressing

*1/3* cup orange juice
*2/3* cup fresh or frozen cranberries (not cooked)
*1* zest of one orange
*1* teaspoon lemon juice
*1/2* teaspoon salt
*1/4* cup peanut oil
*1* tablespoon raw agave nectar

### Instructions

- Place all the ingredients in a food processor for 2 min.

# Grilled Nectarines

*4* whole nectarines
*1/4* cup raw agave nectar
*1/8* teaspoon cinnamon

### Instructions
- Wash nectarines and cut in half, remove seeds
- Mix raw agave and cinnamon on a large plate
- Dip flesh side of the nectarines in the agave mixture to lightly coat.
- On a medium hot grill, place the nectarines flesh side down and close grill lid for 3 minutes
- Remove and place flesh side up

Serves: 8.

# Mango Pineapple Smoothie

*1 1/4* cups Silk Organic Soy Milk (vanilla)
*3/4* cup frozen mango chunks
*1/2* cup frozen pineapple chunks
*1* packet stevia

## Instructions

- Place the ingredients in a blender and blend on high for several minutes. You may have to stop the blender and stir the fruit on the bottom

Serves: 1.

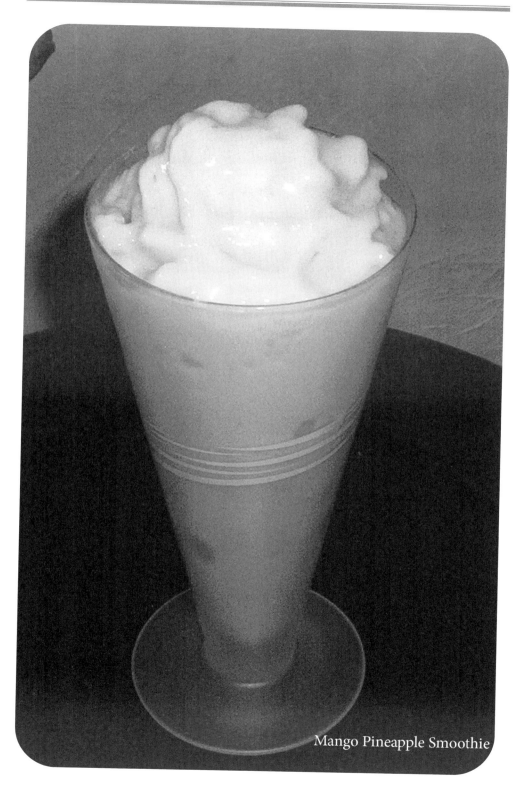

Mango Pineapple Smoothie

# Mixed Berry Smoothie

*1 1/4* cups Silk Organic Soy Milk (vanilla)
*1* cup frozen mixed berries (strawberry, blueberry, raspberry, blackberry)
*1* packet stevia

### Instructions

- Place the ingredients in a blender and blend on high for several minutes. You may have to stop the blender and stir the fruit on the bottom.

This is thick and tastes like a refreshing bowl of sherbet

Serves: 1.

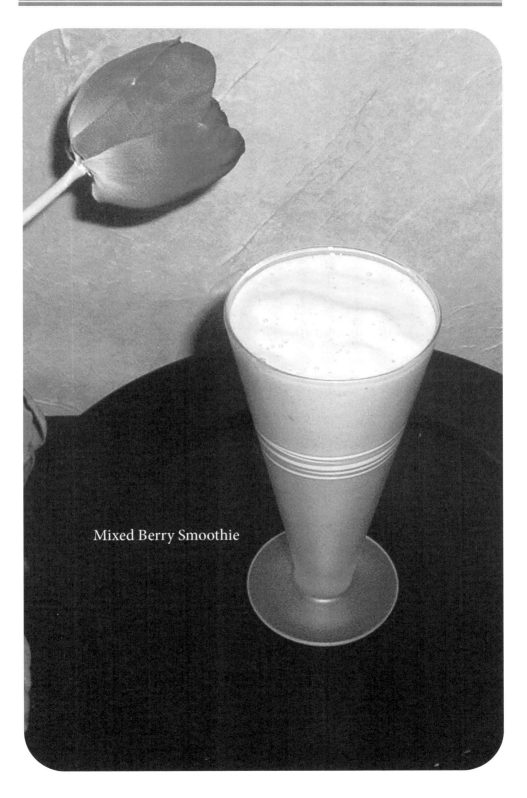

Mixed Berry Smoothie

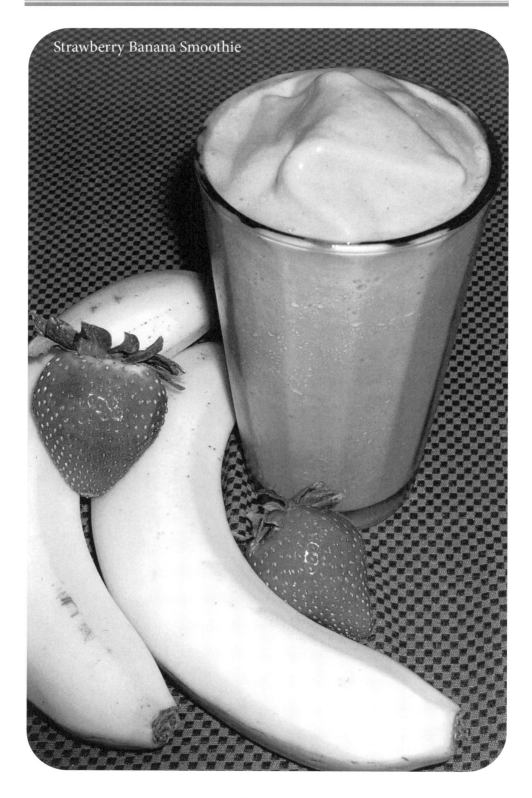

Strawberry Banana Smoothie

# Strawberry Banana Smoothie

*1 1/4* cups Silk Organic Soy Milk (vanilla)
*18* frozen strawberries
*1* cup frozen sliced bananas
*1* packet stevia

## Instructions

- Place the ingredients in a blender and blend on high for several minutes.

You may have to stop the blender and stir the fruit on the bottom.

## Recipe Notes

In order for the smoothie to be thick the fruit must be frozen. Freeze the sliced banana and strawberries together in a Ziploc bag. Do this when you are putting your groceries away... this will insure you have frozen fruit when you are ready to make your smoothie.

Serves: 1.

# Tropical Fruit Bake

*1/2* cup oats (Old Fashioned)
*1/2* cup raw agave nectar
*1* cup whole-grain wheat flour
*2/3* cup coconut oil (organic, extra virgin)
*2/3* cup unsweetened coconut flakes
*2* ounces Macadamia nuts, chopped
*1* 12 oz bag of Frozen Mango Chunks (unsweetened), thawed
*2* 16 oz. bags of Frozen Pineapple chunks (unsweetened), thawed
*4* whole bananas, sliced
*1/2* whole lime, juiced

## *Instructions*

- Preheat oven to 375°
- Select a wide baking dish ..2 to 2 1/2 quart size
- In mixing bowl, add oats, flour, coconut flakes, and macadamia nuts.  Mix together.
- Work the coconut oil into the mixture
- Then stir in the agave nectar. Set aside
- In a large bowl, dump all fruit and lime juice. Toss lightly.
- Place the fruit mixture in the baking dish
- Cover the top of the fruit eenly with the  topping
- Bake for 55 min to an hour. Should be bubbly and brown.

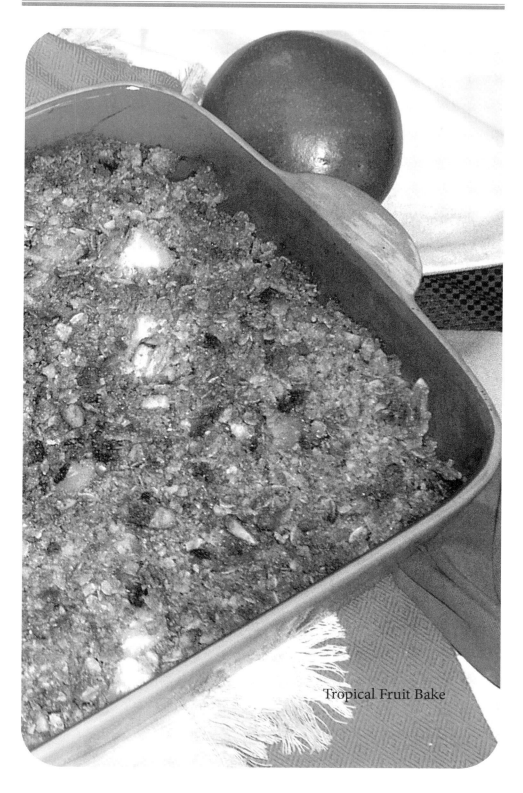

Tropical Fruit Bake

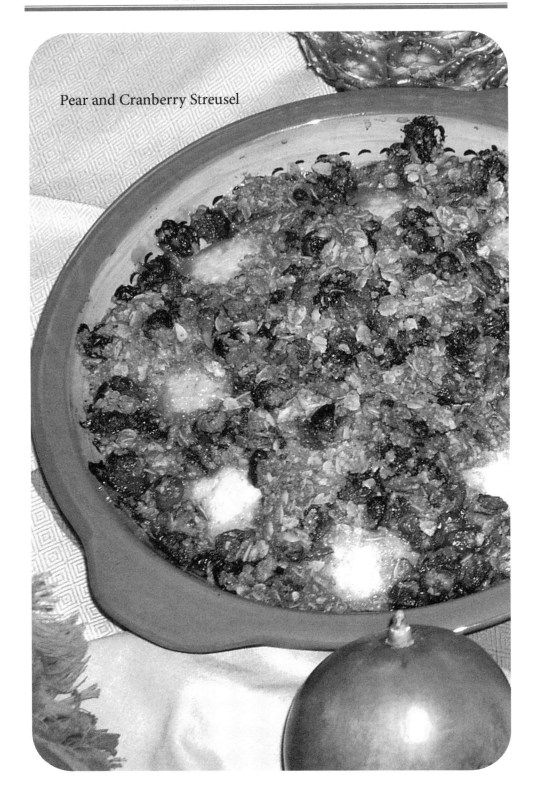

Pear and Cranberry Streusel

# Pear and Cranberry Streusel

*4* whole Bartlett pears
1/8 cup raw agave nectar
*1* tablespoon whole grain, whole wheat flour
*1* teaspoon cinnamon
*1/2* teaspoon nutmeg
Cranberry Streusel Topping (Recipe on following page)

### Instructions

- Preheat oven to 350°
- Peel the pears and cut them in 1/2 through the stem end.
- Use a melon baller to scoop out the cores. Put the pear halves in a large bowl.
- In a small bowl, mix the flour and spices. Stir in the agave nectar
- Coat the pears with the agave nectar mixture
- Put in a peanut oiled baking dish, rounded sides up.
- Prepare the Cranberry Streusel Topping as described in the following recipe.
- Crumble the topping over the pears and bake for 40 to 45 min. or until the topping is crunchy and browned. The pears should be very tender.

### Recipe Notes

*Two 15 ounce canned pears can be substituted for the Bartlett pears. Use the no sugar added, packed in natural pear juice variety.*

# Cranberry Streusel Topping

*1/4* cup peanut oil
*1/2* cup raw agave nectar
*1/2* cup whole grain, whole wheat flour
*1/2* teaspoon kosher salt
*1/2* cup oats (Old Fashioned)
*1/2* cup pecans, chopped
*2* cups cranberries

### Instructions

- In a mixing bowl, mash together the oil and agave, flour and salt with the oats and pecans.
- Toss in the cranberries (you can use frozen or thawed)
- Crumble the topping mixture over fruit in a baking dish.
- Bake at 350° for 40-45 min

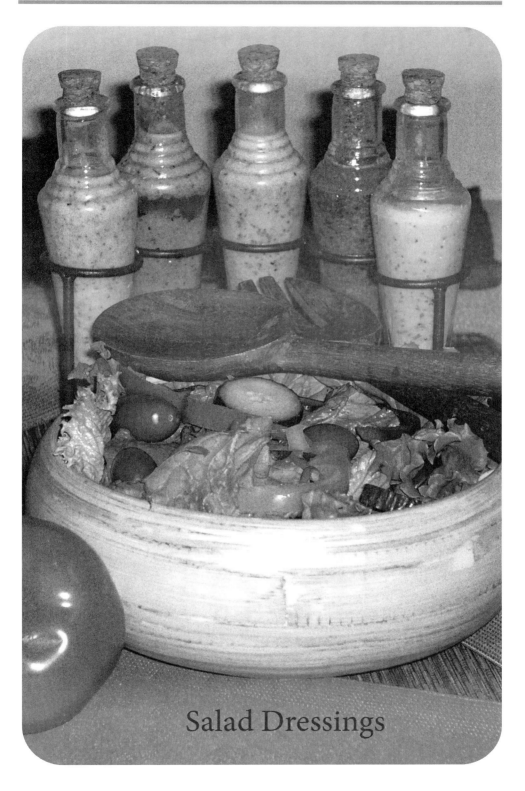

Salad Dressings

# Italian Salad Dressing

*1/4* cup lemon juice

*3* tablespoons water

*1* packet stevia

*3* teaspoons chopped garlic

*2* teaspoons dried onion, minced or powder

*1* teaspoon salt

*1* teaspoon pepper

*2* teaspoons dried parsley

*1* teaspoon dried basil

*1* teaspoon dried oregano

*1/4* teaspoon dried thyme leaves

*1/2* cup olive oil

### Instructions

- Place all ingredients in food processor and blend for 1 minute
- Put in a glass jar and store in the refrigerator. Will keep for two weeks ..if it lasts that long!

# Apple Walnut Salad Dressing

*1/3* cup olive oil
*1/2* teaspoon walnut oil
*1* tablespoon lemon juice
*3* tablespoons apple juice, frozen
*1* package stevia
*1* teaspoon dry mustard
*1* tablespoon minced garlic
*1/4* teaspoon salt
*1/8* teaspoon ground cloves

### Instructions
- Place all ingredients in a food processor and mix on high for 1 minute

### Recipe Notes
The stevia package is an individual sized package sold under the name Sweet Leaf. I have purchased a box of 100 count packets from Wal-Mart. The individual sized packet contains 1/4 teaspoon of stevia.

# Ginger Garlic Japanese Dressing

*3* tablespoons lemon juice
*3* tablespoons peanut oil
*3* tablespoons sesame oil
*3* teaspoons chopped garlic
*1* whole ginger root, 3 in. long peeled and chopped
*5* teaspoons Braggs (Alternative to Soy Sauce)
*1 ½* teaspoons pepper

## Instructions
- Place all ingredients into food processor and blend for 2 minutes
- Keep in refrigerator for 1 week...

## Recipe Notes
*This recipe was created for the Japanese Cabbage Salad.*
*However, it is an excellent dressing for a nice house salad.*

# Sun- Dried Tomato Salad Dressing

*3* tablespoons water
*1* packet stevia
*3* teaspoons chopped garlic
*2* teaspoons dried onion
*1* teaspoon salt
*1* teaspoon pepper
*1* teaspoon dried basil
*1/4* teaspoon dried thyme leaves
*1* tablespoon Italian seasoning
*2* whole sun-dried tomatoes in olive oil
*1/2* cup olive oil

## Instructions

- Place all ingredients in food processor and blend for 1 minute
- Put in a glass jar and store in the refrigerator. Will keep for two weeks...if it lasts that long!

# Green Onion Salad Dressing

*4* whole green onions
*4* tablespoons lemon juice
*1* tablespoon pepper
*1* tablespoon sea salt
*1* tablespoon mustard powder
*1* tablespoon garlic, minced
*1* whole ginger root, about 2 in long, peeled and cut into 4 pieces
*1* whole key lime with seeds removed
*1* cup olive oil

### Instructions

- Wash and cut onions into 2 inch pieces
- Add all the ingredients (Except the Olive Oil) into a food processor. Yes, use the WHOLE key lime.
- Blend for several minutes
- Gradually pour the olive oil through the tube on your food processor, continue blending for several minutes

# Sweet Maple Salad Dressing

*1/4* cup maple syrup
*2* tablespoons lemon juice
*1* teaspoon dry mustard
*1/4* teaspoon salt
*1/4* teaspoon pepper
*1/4* cup olive oil

**Instructions**
- Add all the ingredients to a small bowl and mix thoroughly

# Cilantro Dressing

*1* bunch cilantro leaves
*2* teaspoons minced garlic, jar ok
*2* teaspoons salt
*1* teaspoon pepper
*1* teaspoon cumin
*1/3* cup olive oil
*1* whole lime, juiced

### Instructions
- Place all the ingredients in a food processor and blend for one minute

# Cranberry-Orange Dressing

*1/3* cup orange juice
*2/3* cup fresh or frozen cranberries (not cooked)
*1* zest of one orange
*1* teaspoon lemon juice
*1/2* teaspoon salt
*1/4* cup peanut oil
1 tablespoon raw agave nectar

## Instructions
- Place all the ingredients in a food processor for 2 minutes

## Recipe Notes
This dressing was created for the Pineapple and Mango Fruit Salad. However, it is a delightful dressing for any house salad.

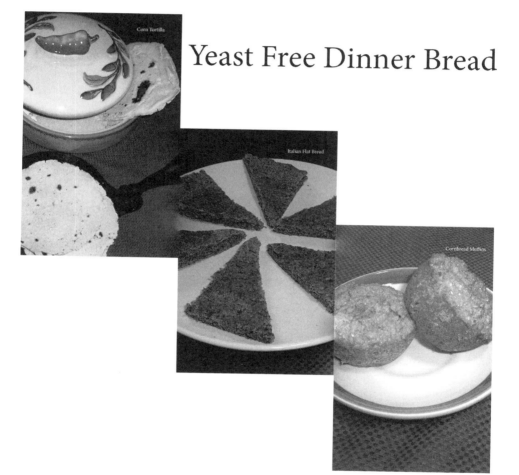

# Yeast Free Dinner Bread

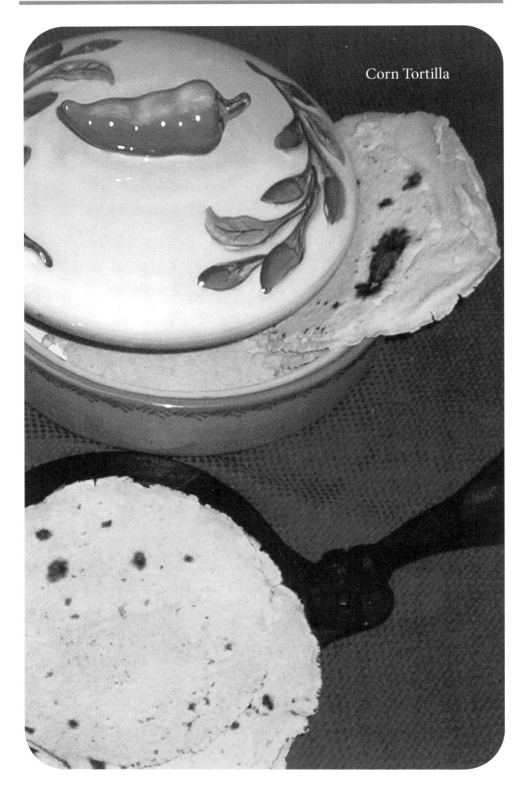

Corn Tortilla

# Corn Tortilla

2 cups Masa corn flour
1 ¼ cups water
1/2 teaspoon salt

## *Instructions*

- Mix the masa, salt and water together in a large bowl. The mixture should stick together...but it should not be too sticky or crumbly. If it is crumbly add 1 tablespoon of water at a time until the desired consistency is accomplished.
- Form into 3 in. balls (a little larger than a golf ball).
- Now its time to press them. You will need a tortilla press and a quart size ziploc bag. (I like to use the zip loc bags instead of wax paper)
- Cut the zip loc bag along the seems...so you will have too square pieces.
- Place the ball in between the ziploc bag pieces on the tortilla press and firmly press down.
- Peel the tortilla away from the ziploc bag
- Cook on a hot griddle, about 2 minutes on each side.

This makes 8-10 tortillas

## *Recipe Notes*

*A tortilla press can be purchased online for about $20..*
*I have also seen them at World Market.*
*Do not use Corn Meal... it is not the same and it will not work.*

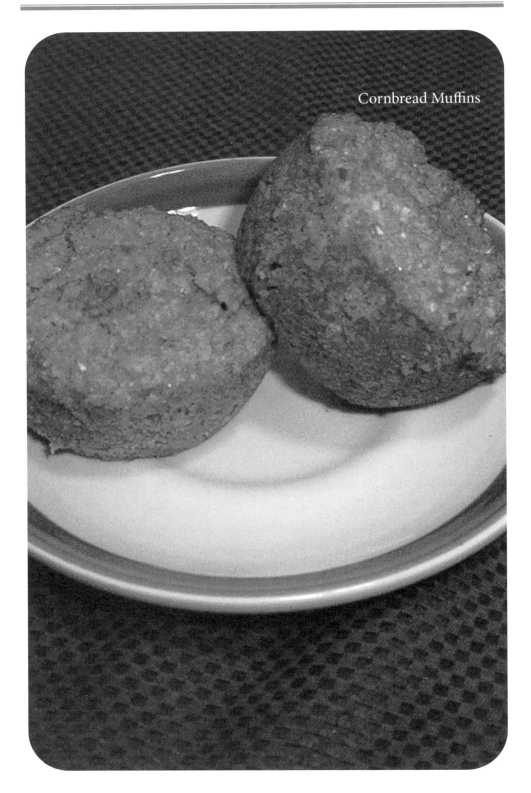

Cornbread Muffins

# Cornbread Muffins

*1* cup GOLDEN ground (milled) flax seed

*1 ½*  cups cornmeal (fine ground)- MED WILL NOT WORK

*1* teaspoon baking soda

*1* teaspoon salt

*1/2* cup raw agave nectar

*1/4* cup olive oil

*1/2* cup soy milk

*1* can corn, drained

### *Instructions*

- Pre heat the oven to 350° and lightly grease muffin pan with a small amount of olive oil.
- In a large bowl, combine ground flax seed, cornmeal, baking soda and salt.
- In food processor, combine drained corn and soy milk, agave nectar and oil oil... puree.
- Pour mixture into the dry ingredients and mix well.
- Spoon the corn bread mixture into the muffin tins, filling the muffins 3/4 full.
- Bake for 15 min. Cool on a rack for 15 minutes before trying to remove from the pan

  Serves: 12.

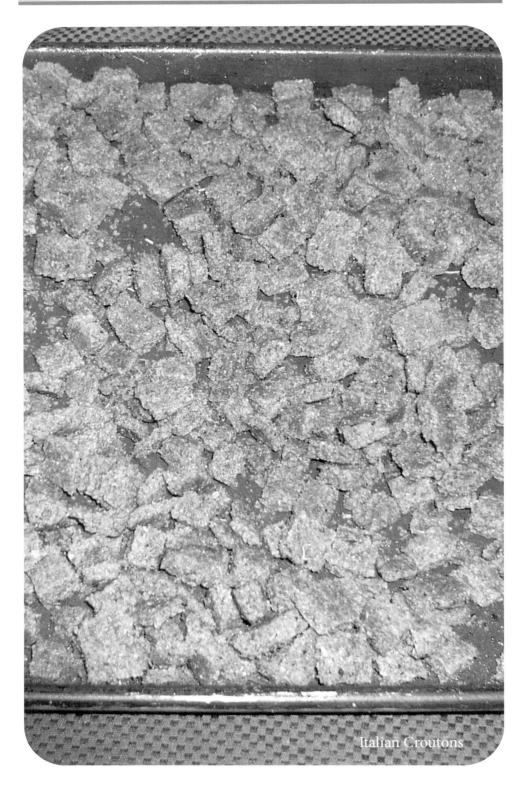

Italian Croutons

# Italian Croutons and Bread Crumbs

Italian Flat bread (recipe follows)
*3/4* cup olive oil
*2* tablespoons garlic powder
*1* tablespoon onion powder
*1* teaspoon Italian seasoning

### Instructions

- Preheat oven to 350°
- Cut the Italian Flat bread into 1/2 inch cubes. (The Italian Flat Bread Recipe makes approximately 8 cups of 1/2 inch cubes)
- Break apart and place in on a cookie sheet in a single layer.
- Combine oil, garlic, onion powder and italian seasoning in a small dish
- Drizzle the oil mixture over the bread cubes. Lightly toss.
- Bake for 25-30 min tossing every 5 min. Croutons should be dry and toasty.

To make Bread Crumbs

- Put desired amount of toasted croutons in the blender and poof... bread Crumbs :)

### Recipe Notes
*To keep longer, freeze in small plastic baggies.*

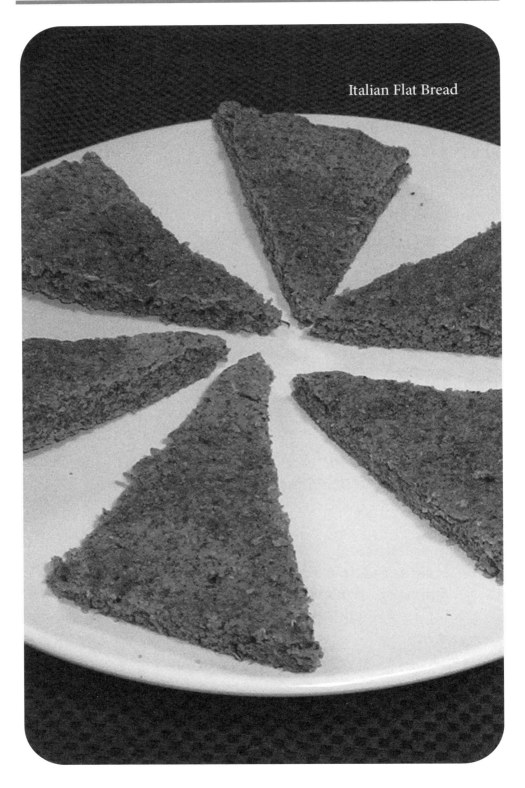

Italian Flat Bread

# Italian Flat Bread

*2* cups whole grain, whole wheat flour
*1* cup Milled Flax seed (flour)
*1/2* teaspoon baking soda
*1* teaspoon fennel seed
*1/2* teaspoon dried basil
*1/4* teaspoon dried oregano
*1/4* teaspoon dried thyme leaves
*1/2* teaspoon garlic powder
*1/2* teaspoon onion powder
*1 ½* cups warm water
*1* teaspoon lemon juice
*2* tablespoons olive oil, divided use
*1/2* teaspoon salt, to taste

### Instructions

- Pre heat oven to 350° Oil a sheet pan with 1 TBSP of olive oil
- Combine flour, ground flax seed, soda, and all the spices in a large bowl.
-  In a separate bowl combine water and lemon juice.
- Add lemon water to the dry ingredients and mix with your hands until well blended.
- Use 1 tablespoon of oil to grease a sheet pan.  Press into the sheet pan and bake for 20 min
- Brush top with 1 tablespoon of olive oil and sprinkle with salt

# Whole Grain Crackers

*1* cup whole grain, whole wheat flour
*1* cup spelt flour
*1* teaspoon salt
*1* teaspoon garlic powder
*1* teaspoon onion powder
*1/3* cup olive oil
*1/3* cup water, plus 2-3 tablespoons

## Instructions

- Preheat oven to 375°
- Combine flours, salt garlic and onion powders and then work the olive oil into the flour.
- Then add the water while you work the dough with the other hand... until it is not dry nor sticky.
- Press very thin on to a cookie sheet and cut into 1.5 inch squares.
- Bake at 375° for 20-25 min or until crispy but not burnt.

Serves: 6.

# Whole Grain Pizza Crust

*2* cups whole grain, whole wheat flour
*1/3* cup olive oil
*1* cup water
*1* teaspoon Italian seasoning
*1/2* teaspoon salt
*1* teaspoon fennel seed
*1/4* teaspoon garlic powder
*1* tablespoon olive oil for pan

### Instructions

- Mix flour, salt and seasonings in a large bowl.
- Add oil and work into the flour well, until the oil and flour are combined.
- As you are mixing the dough with your hands, slowly add 1 cup of water. This should form a well behaved dough.
- Knead until smooth.. If too dry add small amounts of water(1 tablespoon at a time). If it is too sticky, add 1 tablespoon of flour at a time.
- Press into a greased cookie sheet to make one large pizza or roll out into individual sized pizzas. You can use a tortilla press to make small pizzas. Makes 6-8 individual sized pizzas

For best results bake on a pizza stone at 375°, until the crust is crispy. This takes about 30 minutes with toppings.

# Whole-Wheat Flat Bread

2 cups whole grain, whole wheat flour
1 cup Milled Flax seed (flour)
1 ½ cups warm water
2 tablespoons olive oil
1/2 teaspoon salt
2 teaspoons flax seeds

## Instructions

- Pre heat oven to 350°. Oil a 13" X 9" pan with 1 TBSP of olive oil
- Combine flour, ground flax seed in a large bowl.
- Add water to the dry ingredients and mix with your hands until well blended. Press into the 13"X9" pan.
- Sprinkle with Flax seeds and press into the top.
- Bake for 20 minutes
- While hot, brush top with 1 TBSP of olive oil and sprinkle with salt

## Recipe Notes

*This bread is not soft like the Italian Bread. It is great to dip in a garlic, red pepper olive oil.*

Serves: 8.

# Whole-Wheat Tortilla

*2* cups whole grain, whole wheat flour
*1* teaspoon salt
*1/3* cup olive oil
*2/3* cup warm water

## Instructions

- Mix flour and salt together in a large bowl.
- Add oil and work into the flour well, until all flour and oil are combined.
- Then slowly add 2/3 cup water as you are mixing the dough with your hands. This should form a well behaved dough.
- Knead until smooth...usually takes a couple of min. If too dry add small amounts of water (1 tablespoon).
- Divide in half four times, making 8 equal balls.
- Cover with plastic wrap and let sit for 20-30 minutes.
- On a smooth surface, lay out a piece of wax paper and place a ball in the center. Place another piece of wax paper on top.
- Use a rolling pin to press tortillas into mostly round shapes. This takes a little practice. Don't expect perfectly round tortillas the first time you attempt this!
- Cook on a hot griddle or frying pan. Cook 2 minutes on each side.

## Recipe Notes

*Using a Tortilla press makes this recipe a breeze!*
*Simply put the ball of tortilla dough in the center of the press and push down. Then cook them on a hot griddle.*

# Refreshing Beverages

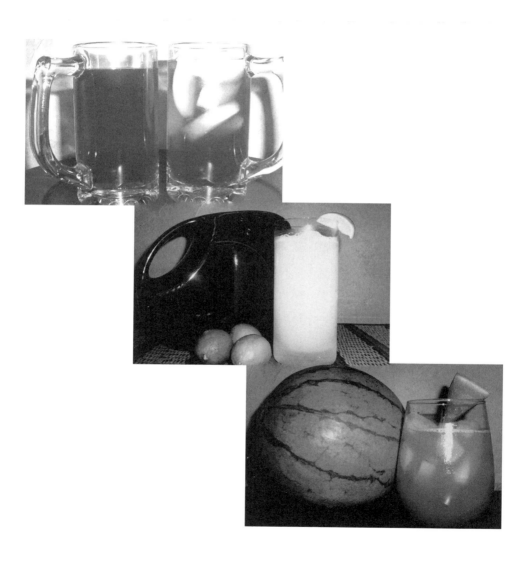

# Blueberry Pomegranate Tea

*12* tea bags of Celestial Seasonings Wild Berry Zinger
*4* packets stevia
*1/2* cup pomegranate w/wild blueberry juice
*6* cups water, boiling

## Instructions

- Place the tea bags in a heat resistant container, stevia and juice.
- Pour the boiling water over the bags and cover, let steep for 6 min's.
- Great hot or poured over ice.
- Refrigerate leftovers for a quick refreshing cold drink or microwave a cup for a tranquil moment

Serves: 4.

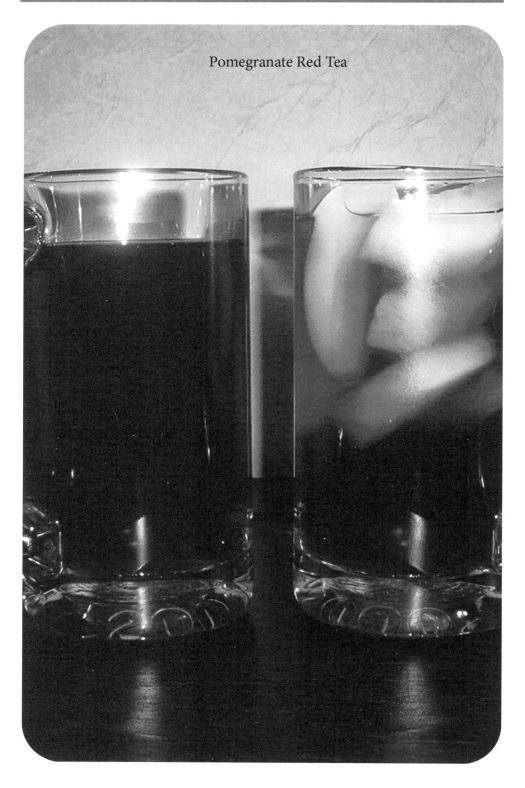

Pomegranate Red Tea

# Pomegranate Red Tea

*12* tea bag from Celestial Seasonings Moroccan Pomegranate Red Tea
*4* packets stevia
*1/3* cup pomegranate juice
*6* cups boiling water

## Instructions

- Place 12 tea bags in a heat resistant container add stevia and pomegranate juice, pour in 6 cups of boiling water.
- Cover and let steep for 6 minutes.
- Remove bags, stir and drink either hot or over ice...delicious.
- Refrigerate leftovers

## Recipe Notes

*This makes a refreshing glass of iced tea or put a cup in the microwave for a convenient cup of hot tea.*

Serves: 4.

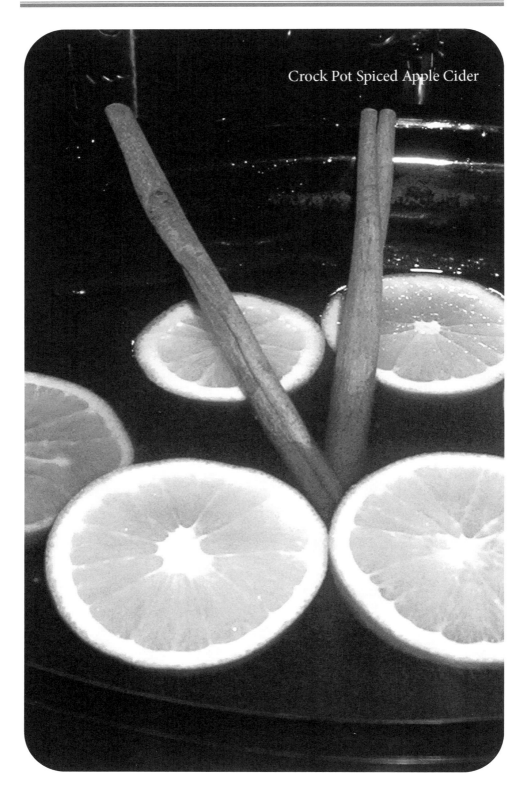

Crock Pot Spiced Apple Cider

# Crock Pot Spiced Apple Cider

*1* gallon natural apple cider
*3* large mexican cinnamon sticks or 6 small
*10* whole cloves
*20* whole all spice
*1* whole orange, sliced

### Instructions

- Place all of the ingredients into a large crock pot, start out on high for the first hour uncovered...then turn down to low and let simmer all day...(at least 4 hours)
- Remove cinnamon sticks and with a slotted spoon, remove all spice and cloves.

Serve hot... Makes the house smell so wonderful !! Put the leftovers back in the apple cider jug with a funnel. Refrigerate ...then pour into a mug and microwave until hot...will keep for up to a week.

Serves: 8.

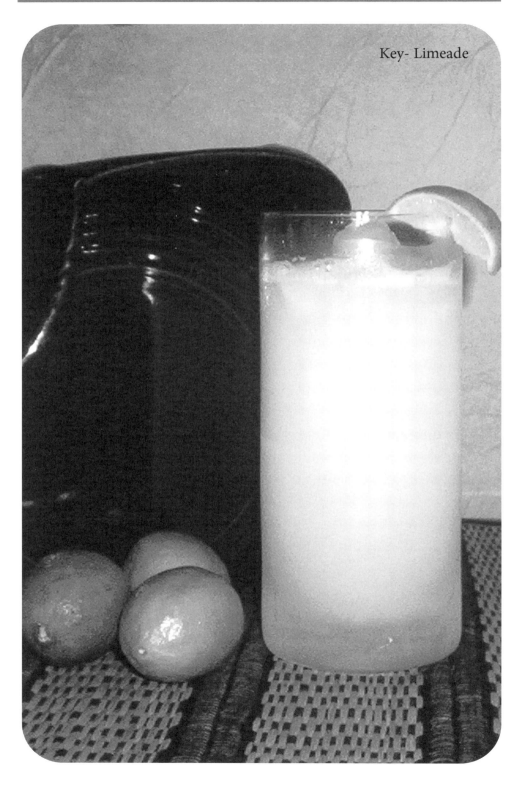

Key- Limeade

# Key- Limeade

*6* whole key limes cut in half
*6* cups water
*10* packages stevia, small individual packets

### Instructions

- In a blender combine, the key limes (seeds and all), 2 cups of water and 10 packages of stevia. Blend on high for 1 minute.
- Strain into a pitcher and add the remaining 4 cups of water.

Serve this refreshing drink over ice and garnish with a slice of key lime

Serves: 4.

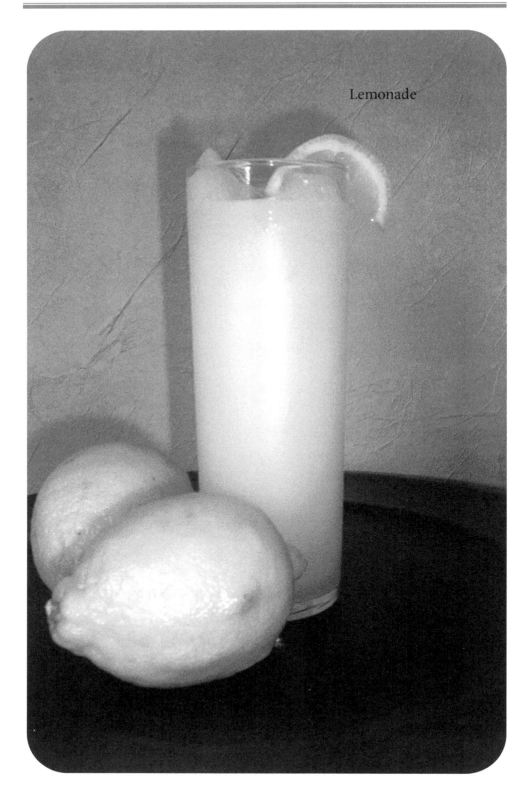

Lemonade

# Lemonade

*2* medium lemons
*10* packages stevia
*1* whole lemon, juiced
*6* cups water

### Instructions

- Remove the ends of 2 lemons, cut into 6 pieces each and put all in the blender along with 1 1/2 cups of water and 10 packages of stevia and the juice of 1 lemon. Blend for 1 min
- Then strain into pitcher, add remaining 4 ½ cups of water and stir well. Serve over ice.

I like to make two batches, that way I'll have plenty for a couple of days

Serves: 6.

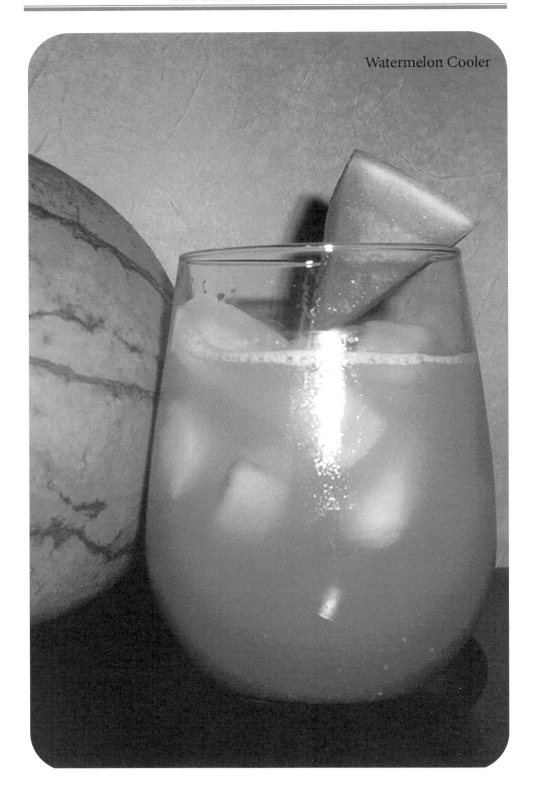

Watermelon Cooler

# Watermelon Cooler

*1* small seedless watermelon, needs to yield 8 cups
*4* cups water
*4* packets stevia

### Instructions
- Remove rind from watermelon and cut into pieces.
- In 3 batches add watermelon 1/2 way up the blender and add 1 1/3 cups of water and 1 packet of stevia blend for at least 1 min to completely puree.
- Place blended watermelon in a pitcher and repeat the process.
- In the last batch add 2 packets of stevia

This is so delicious....serve over ice...truly a treat in the middle of winter and even better in the summer

Serves: 6.

# About the Authors

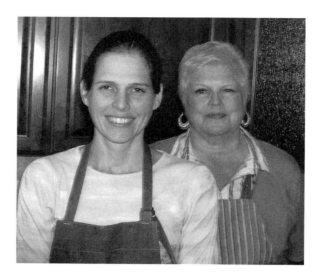

**Grace Bass** is the mother of four children and wife of Rev. Patrick Bass, Pastor of New Life Church of Tempe in Tempe, Arizona. She was born and raised in south and central Texas. She is currently enrolled at Western Governors University as a full time student and homeschools two of their children.

**Lynda (Louscher) Anderson** is the mother of Grace Bass and wife of Lyle Anderson. She was born and raised in Lake Park, Iowa. For 15 years, Lynda was the Founder and CEO of Des Laurier Perfumes, Inc.  While enjoying retirement, she sits on the Board of Directors for the Lago Vista Players Association; she enjoys cooking and serving her community in Lago Vista, Texas.

# Works Cited

"Agave Nectar." <http://en.wikipedia.org/wiki/Agave_nectar>.

Barnes. Barnes Notes. 1Barnes' Notes, Electronic Database. Copyright (C) 1997 by Biblesoft.

"Fats & Cholesterol." Harvard School of Public Health. Harvard School. Fall 2007 <http://www.hsph.harvard.edu/now/>.

Hendry, Joene. "Experts Weigh in: Will Trans Fat Bans Affect ObesityTrends?" DOC News os 4 (2007): 1. American Diabetes Association. Fall 2007.

"Honey." Fall 2007 <http://en.wikipedia.org/wiki/Honey>.

"Olive Oil." <http://en.wikipedia.org/wiki/Olive_oil>.

"Our 2006 Diet and Lifestyle Recommendations." 2006. American Heart Association. Fall 2007 <http://www.americanheart.org/presenter.jhtml?identifier=851>.

"Stevia." Fall 2007 <http://en.wikipedia.org/wiki/Stevia>.

"Sugarcane." <http://en.wikipedia.org/wiki/Sugar_cane>.

Thompson Chain-Reference Study Bible. Indianopolis: B.B. KIRKBRIDE BIBLE COMPANY, INC., 2000.

Towns, Elmer L. Fasting for Spiritual Break Through. Ventura: Regal Books, 1996. 1-251.

# Fasting Journal

In the Gospel of John chapter 21 it is recorded that the disciples fished all night and caught nothing. In the morning, Jesus appeared to them and told them to cast their net on the other side of the boat. The disciples were no doubt tired. However, when they decided to give it a try, a miracle occurred!! Multitudes of fish were caught, so much so they could not draw in the nets! When they dragged the nets to the shore, Jesus told them to bring the fish they had now caught. It is recorded in verse 11 that there was 153 fish!! Think about this, someone had to count the fish! And then it was written down!

While you are fasting and drawing closer to God, let this encourage you to count the many blessings God has given to you and write them down!!

| Length of Fast: | Date Started: | Date Ended: |
|---|---|---|
| *Special Testimony:* | | |
| | | |
| | | |
| | | |
| | | |

| Length of Fast: | Date Started: | Date Ended: |
|---|---|---|
| *Special Testimony:* | | |
| | | |
| | | |
| | | |
| | | |

| Length of Fast: | Date Started: | Date Ended: |
|---|---|---|
| *Special Testimony*: | | |
| | | |
| | | |
| | | |
| | | |

| Length of Fast: | Date Started: | Date Ended: |
|---|---|---|
| *Special Testimony*: | | |
| | | |
| | | |
| | | |
| | | |

| Length of Fast: | Date Started: | Date Ended: |
|---|---|---|
| *Special Testimony*: | | |
| | | |
| | | |
| | | |
| | | |

| Length of Fast: | Date Started: | Date Ended: |
|---|---|---|
| *Special Testimony*: | | |
| | | |
| | | |
| | | |
| | | |

# Alphabetical Index